Charles H. Schaible

First Help in Accidents

Charles H. Schaible

First Help in Accidents

ISBN/EAN: 9783337294410

Printed in Europe, USA, Canada, Australia, Japan

Cover: Foto ©Lupo / pixelio.de

More available books at **www.hansebooks.com**

FIRST HELP IN ACCIDENTS:

BEING

A SURGICAL GUIDE,

IN THE ABSENCE OR BEFORE THE ARRIVAL OF MEDICAL ASSISTANCE,

FOR THE USE OF THE PUBLIC,

ESPECIALLY

FOR THE MEMBERS OF BOTH THE MILITARY AND NAVAL SERVICES,
VOLUNTEERS AND TRAVELLERS, ETC.

BY

CHARLES H. SCHAIBLE, M.D., Ph. D.

ROYAL MILITARY ACADEMY, WOOLWICH;
EXAMINER IN THE GERMAN LANGUAGE AND LITERATURE IN THE
UNIVERSITY OF LONDON;

*Member of the Council, Licentiate and Examiner in Natural History and Physiology
in the College of Preceptors; Corresponding Member of the Association of
Medical Officers for the Advancement of Public Medicine of Baden;
and of other foreign Societies.*

"Nihil homines propius Deo accedunt, quam salutem hominibus dando."—Cicero, pro Q. Ligarin.

LONDON:
ROBERT HARDWICKE, 192, PICCADILLY;
AND ALL BOOKSELLERS.

Alphabetical List of Chief Sections.

Asphyxia, 161.
Bad Air, Suffocation by, 166.
Bad Food, 158.
Bleeding, 43.
Blood Vessels, 33.
Broken Bones, 103.
Bruises, 72.
Burns, 75.
Choking, 134.
Cold, Effects of, Frozen Limbs, 82.
Contusions, 72.
Death, Signs of, 186.
Dislocations, 90.
Dog-Bite, 156.
Drowning, 165.
Drunkenness, 153.
Exhaustion on Marches, 217.
Faintness on Marches, 216.
Foreign Bodies in Throat, Gullet, Air-passage, 134.
Fractures, 103.
Gases, Suffocation by, 166.
Hanging, Suffocation by, 162.
Heat, Effect of, 86.
Insect-bite, 155.
Litters, 197.

Marches, Accidents on. 190.
Poisoning, 141.
  By Acids, 148.
  „ Alkalies, 149.
  „ Metallic Poisons, 150.
  „ Vegetable Poisons, 151.
  „ Narcotic Poisons, 151.
  „ Opium, 151.
  „ Prussic Acid, 153.
  „ Alcohol, 153.
Scalds, 75.
Snake-bite, 156.
Sprains, 90.
Strangulation, 162.
Suffocation, 161.
Sunstroke, 86.
Swallowing of noxious things, 159.
Transport of Patients, 190.
Vapours inhaled, 154.
Walking, Hygienic Rules for, 213.
Wounds, Dressing of, 9.
Wounds, Treatment of, 53.
Wounds, Poisoned, 156.

PREFACE.

MY frequent intercourse with· gentlemen of the military profession has convinced me that a short and clear surgical Guide for the treatment of Accidents, to which they are especially exposed, would be a welcome contribution to a soldier's library, and has led me to write the present work, which I originally intended for their use exclusively. Thinking, however, that the book might be of some utility to the public at large, I have been induced to give it a more general character. Although various very useful books of a somewhat similar kind have already been issued in this country, yet I believe that none of them have exactly the same scope as the work which I now venture to submit to the public. Some of them are more limited in their objects, treating only of certain classes of accidents; others are more extensive, and complete treatises on all kinds of occurrences that may happen in a quiet household. As my object has been to produce a manual for the use not only of the domestic circle, but also of the soldier, sailor, volunteer, and traveller, explaining briefly and clearly what ought to be done by non-professional persons, *before the arrival, or in the absence of a medical man,* for the relief of those who are suffering from various *serious* accidents, I trust that my work will be found to supply a desideratum in this department of literature.

Being a foreigner, and having never practised Medicine and Surgery in England, in which I have not resided many years, I am conscious that in presenting to the public a book of this kind, in a country famous for its eminent surgeons, I may appear to be somewhat bold, especially as I am well aware of the numerous deficiencies and imperfections in style and matter, which will meet the eye of even a friendly critic. For the language and style I may venture to claim some indulgence; in extenuation of the defects, attributable to want of sufficient leisure to perfect the book, I would simply plead my ardent desire to employ my few leisure hours in the service of the community that has hospitably welcomed me. If the end I have had in view—the diffusion of knowledge that may add to the comfort or save the life of some suffering fellow-creature—be attained, in however small a degree, I shall not regret having followed the maxim, "*bis dat, qui cito dat,*" in preference to delaying the appearance of the work, by frequent alterations and revisions.

I feel it my pleasant duty to express my great obligations to my friend, William Newman, Esq., M.D. Lond., of Stamford, for his valuable assistance in revising this little volume, and for the numerous improvements which it has received from his pen.

CHARLES H. SCHAIBLE.

London, *September*, 1864.

CONTENTS

INTRODUCTION.

Immediate help important—Presence of mind depends upon knowing what and how to do—Helplessness of injured soldiers on battle-field—Usefulness of an elementary surgical instruction to soldiers—Popular medicine objectionable; popular elementary surgery, with practical exercises, valuable, fit for school teaching and beneficial to society—Sanitary soldiers' companies in Germany; their instruction in dressing and transport; such knowledge useful to civilians as well as soldiers—The highly-trained medical man the only person qualified to teach such knowledge .... *page* xvii

GENERAL REMARKS.

Coolness and presence of mind necessary—Immediate treatment, rules for—Yet professional aid should be had, if possible...*page* 1

CHAPTER I.

DRESSING OF WOUNDS.

§ 1. Articles needed for Immediate Dressings—Water, Sponges, Flannel, Lint, Oil-Silk, Gutta-Percha Tissue, Plasters, Linen, Splints and Bandages—List of articles which might be carried in package .... *page* 9

§ 2. Subsequent Dressings—Cold and Heat: their application as local agents—Evaporating Lotions — Ice — Irrigation — Immersion. Heat: Dry; Moist—Water Dressing—Fomentations. Poultices: Mustard Poultices —Leeches .... *page* 20

§ 3. Stimulants: when and how to use them—Coffee—Brandy............................*page* 30

CHAPTER II.

BLEEDING: SOURCE AND ARRESTING OF.

§ 1. Blood-Vessels — Circulation of Blood — Enumeration and brief description of the principal arteries and veins; their course and

CONTENTS. xi

arrangement—The points specially mentioned where compression may be practised ... *page* 33

§ 2. How to arrest Bleeding—By employment of Cold—Pressure, local or distant: by fingers or tourniquet—Position or Ligature...... *page* 43

CHAPTER III.

WOUNDS: THEIR VARIETIES AND TREATMENT.

General plan of Treatment—Incised Wounds—Treatment of—Modes of Healing—Treatment of Punctured Wounds or Pricks—Treatment of Lacerated or Torn Wounds—Treatment of Contused Wounds and of Gunshot Wounds—Subsequent Treatment of Wounds—Astringent applications, &c. *page* 53

CHAPTER IV.

BRUISES AND CONTUSIONS.

Moisture and Rest—Leeches .... *page* 72

CHAPTER V.

BURNS AND SCALDS.

Different degrees of—Absence of Pain a bad Symptom — Locality influences result — Applications, Dry or Moist — Warm and Stimulating Dressings to be preferred —Lime under the Eyelids—Treatment of Chemical Agents—Their action on the Skin—Antidotes for .... *page* 75

CHAPTER VI

EFFECTS OF COLD AND HEAT—FROZEN LIMBS, SUN-STROKE, ETC.

§ 1. Effects of Cold—The return to normal heat in room and dressings must be very gradual, or Mortification may result — Protection against Frostbite .... *page* 83

§ 2. Effects of Heat—Sunstroke—Bleeding to be avoided — Support and Stimulants given .... *page* 86

CHAPTER VII.

SPRAINS—DISLOCATIONS.

Definitions of these terms—*Sprains* need rest, cold application, and subsequently support—Often tedious in recovery. *Dislocations*—Symptoms of—General Remarks—Special Forms—Lower Jaw Dislocated—Reduction of—Shoulder and Hip Joints may be thus Injured—The necessary Treatment—Displacement of Cartilage in Knee Joint—Reduction of .... *page* 90

CHAPTER VIII.

FRACTURES, OR BROKEN BONES.

Distinction between Fractures and Dislocations—Fractures are Simple or Compound—Points to be had in view in Treatment—Directions for applying Splints, Bandages, &c.—Special Fractures noticed—Ribs, Collar-Bone, Upper and Fore Arm, Thigh, Leg—Bones of Face and Lower Jaw .... *page* 103

CHAPTER IX.

OF THE LODGMENT OF FOREIGN BODIES IN THE THROAT, IN THE GULLET, OR IN THE AIR PASSAGES.

The Localities which foreign Bodies may reach—Mode of dealing with them............... *page* 134

CHAPTER X.

OF POISONING.

General Rules of Symptoms which may excite the suspicion of Poison—Division of Poisons into Classes, and the Subdivisions of these Classes—Treatment of Poisoning—General and Special Rules—Animal Poisons—Modes of Reception into System—Modes of Treatment .... *page* 141

CHAPTER XI.

OF SUFFOCATION.

How caused—The Treatment of different Forms —Due to Hanging or Strangulation.—To

Drowning, or to Exposure to Narcotic or Irrespirable Gases — Results of Impure Atmosphere even in minor degree—Rules issued by the Royal Humane Society and the Royal National Life-boat Institution ... *page* 161

CHAPTER XII.

OF THE SIGNS OF REAL DEATH.

Enumeration of these Indications and their comparative Value—Practical Bearings *page* 186

CHAPTER XIII.

OF TRANSPORT OF INJURED PERSONS AND OF INVALIDS.

The means to be employed for this purpose *page* 190

§ 1. When no special means are available, human arms and strength may yet be employed .... *page* 191

§ 2. When litters can be obtained or constructed—Forms of—Muskets may be used for this purpose, &c. .... *page* 197

§ 3. Vehicles may be Impressed—How to use them to most advantage—How to Transport Injured Persons in Railways .... *page* 203

§ 3. Animals may be Useful—How best to turn them to good purpose .... *page* 211

CHAPTER XIV.

HYGIENIC RULES FOR WALKING AND FOR MARCHES—ACCIDENTS WHICH MAY HAPPEN TO SOLDIERS ON MARCH.

Clothing in its Details—Weight, how to Carry—Division of Time occupied in Exercise, &c.—Faintness, Exhaustion, &c., during a March .... *page* 213

CHAPTER XV.

RESUMÉ OF DIRECTIONS FOR THE TREATMENT OF SEVERE ACCIDENTS OR INJURIES.

Examination and Position of Patient—First steps in cases of Bleeding, Wounds, Spraining, Fracture—Foreign bodies in the Eyes—Alphabetical List of all the Chief Sections of the Book, to facilitate information ... *page* 219

INTRODUCTION.

IT is the duty of every man to help a fellow-creature in case of need. But, in order that this may be done effectually, it is indispensable that a knowledge of the best courses of action should be possessed.

If an accident happens, attended by a considerable flow of blood, the sympathies of the bystanders are at once aroused; they are anxious to assist the sufferer, and, with presence of mind and calmness, they may afford much valuable aid until the services of a surgeon can be obtained. But this presence of mind and calm judgment are the result of knowing *how efficient help may be given.* Life itself not unfrequently depends on the first treatment of the injured person, since medical aid may be long in reaching him, especially in secluded dwellings, during military operations, and in vessels at sea.

In reports from the field of battle, it is by no means uncommon to find complaints that many unfortunate men have been left a considerable time, it may even be for days, without having had their wounds properly dressed. The general impression would seem to be that surgical dressings are so complicated and tedious, that it is not possible to apply even the first bandage without professional aid, or to give efficient protection, at least for a time, in the case of accidents attended with complete personal helplessness; and yet much may be done by a little well-applied knowledge.

Soldiers are trained to inflict injuries on

the enemy, to avoid needless exposure of their own persons: why may they not also be enabled to take care of their comrades when wounds are inflicted? Not only might instruction of this kind be easily and quickly imparted, but its possession would give pleasure and self-reliance to the combatant. Will he not go into action with increased confidence when assured that, if a quick and glorious death be not the immediate consequence of some severe wound, he will meet with speedy assistance, and with such aid as the injury may demand?

In the Homeric ages, kings and generals vied in their efforts to afford help to their wounded warriors: why should our modern soldiery prove themselves less competent or less humane?

For the speedy treatment of some special accidents, such as suffocation occasioned by drowning or hanging, various forms of poisoning, &c., rules have been laid down, in this country, by societies and writers, and on the Continent, by the sanitary police; but in most cases this has been done with regard to one particular class of accidents only. It would seem, then, that there is room for further instruction, not only in selected cases, but also in the treatment and appliances necessary for accidents or injuries of daily occurrence. How few even of the educated classes are competent to direct or put in practice the necessary proceedings!

That it is for many reasons unwise, if not absolutely dangerous, to attempt to give popular directions for the treatment of internal diseases, those cases alone excepted where immediate action is imperative, is an opinion that has been for years steadily gaining ground among men of science: works on *popular medicine* have consequently been valued according to their deserts. It is otherwise, however, with *popular surgery*—the term being used in a limited sense, and referring to those early manipulations and applications which, in the absence of qualified surgical assistance, are of such extreme value where local injuries have occurred.

The time is, we trust, not far distant when the study of physiology as applied to the preservation of personal health, and of surgery so far as it may be necessary for the immediate treatment of minor casualties, will enter into the curriculum of ordinary education, and fill up some hours which are now devoted to far less important objects.

The conditions of health and life, so dear to every one, would be better understood and recognized, and the whole community would directly benefit by the extension of such thoroughly useful knowledge. There is no foundation for the objections that there would be great difficulty in imparting the required information, or that much time would be occupied in communicating it.

The system of manipulations and bandaging, sufficient to meet all ordinary requirements—such as that recommended by the celebrated Dr. Mayor, now nearly half a century ago—would be learnt by an attentive person in a very few days. If the theoretical directions as to dressing, bandaging, &c., be combined with practical exercises, either on the living body or on duly prepared models, the knowledge would prove more precise and more available when suddenly called for:

> "Segnius irritant animos demissa per aures,
> Quam quæ sunt oculis subjecta fidelibus."

In some countries of Europe—Germany, for example—soldiers in selected companies are now instructed in the transport of the wounded, and in the early dressings of the simpler forms of wounds. To aid their instructors, Dr. Beck, a distinguished and experienced military surgeon of Baden, has written a small work, to which the author of the present book cheerfully acknowledges his obligation for certain chapters of this work. It is of paramount importance that military men should possess such elementary knowledge; yet, though less frequently, private life has its accidents and its sufferers, and therefore the requisite directions should be generally known. Instruction of this kind would undoubtedly be most properly given towards the close of the school studies, and as the pupils are drafted off one by one to their separate localities and callings, they would carry with them a tangible and very valuable store of minor surgical acquirement.

To the highly-trained surgeon alone could this task of education with advantage be committed. None can so well popularize a scientific subject as those who are thoroughly at home in what they teach; none so well mark out the salient points of a journey as those who have traversed paths parallel to the main road. Thus the surgeon would add the calling of teacher to his daily routine, and prove his labours of essential service in dispelling prejudices, and in diffusing far and wide knowledge of the highest utility.

FIRST HELP IN ACCIDENTS.

GENERAL REMARKS.

IN order successfully to meet the various requirements of a case of accidental injury or of sudden seizure, it is imperative that the helper bring, to aid him in the task, the two conditions of *coolness* and *presence of mind*. It may be at once conceded that all do not in a like degree possess these qualities; but it is none the less thoroughly true that, existing it may be only in a minor degree, they may by the majority of persons be successfully cultivated and developed. If the bystander be flurried and uncertain, he will but increase the misery he so much desires to remedy, and his services, dictated by the best motives, will have lost much of their value. Thought and will must be concentrated on the work before him; the patient in his own special individuality must be lost sight of, and the hurt, whatever it may be, must receive the fullest and closest consideration. Deep and thorough sympathy with the fellow-creature is quite compatible with an apparent neglect of the feelings of the sufferer; and an indifference to querulous complaint may be well pardoned, when the whole attention is absorbed by the tending of some positive damage. Quietly, calmly, and thoroughly must the necessary inquiries be made, and the appropriate treatment carried out. A course of action once determined on should not be deviated from, either in misplaced pity for the injured person, or in deference to the objections of some less clear-headed looker-on.

To speak, in the first instance, of the immediate treatment of some one who may have met with severe local injury, the following rules may be laid down without hesitation in general terms. Separate and succeeding chapters will deal more clearly with the special directions necessary for particular wounds :—

1. Ascertain at once the history and the place of injury—and this by a few terse, clear questions—

    (a) From the patient himself, if he be sensible and able to speak; but if he be insensible,

    (b) From the bystanders—if any were near : make out what they have seen, what they know, but on no account waste time in listening to details unconnected with and irrelevant to the point at issue.

2. If the patient be insensible, place him on the ground or floor, lying rather

over to or directly on one side, and with the head slightly raised, so that it be placed on the same level with the rest of the body; this will tend to his breathing more easily than if he be placed flat on the back. Then remove necktie, collar, &c., and unbutton or split open any clothing pressing tightly upon the neck, chest, or abdomen.

3. As a restorative the face and chest may be sprinkled with cold water, and then wiped dry; some cold water may be drunk if the power of swallowing be present; but do not hastily pour stimulants down the throat unless there be clear evidence that they are needed.

4. Nor, acting on the opposite principle, allow some officious individual to bleed, in the view of preventing inflammation, a man whose danger

lies for the present at least far more in the shock of the injury, and in impending collapse.

5. Examine one by one the limbs—their prominent parts you may examine by touch and grasping with very little movement of the whole frame: if there be bleeding, note from whence it comes, following the directions given further on; and look to any change of outline, swelling, &c., in the extremities.

6. If there be distinct local injury let it be treated on the ordinary plans, and with such appliances as you have at hand. Having seen to this.

7. Then attend to the removing of the patient. (See chapter on Transport.) On no account, if there be severe injury to head or any part of frame, allow him to mount a horse, or to sit

upright in a vehicle, but let him lie down as thoroughly as possible. Walking also should be avoided on the same grounds.

8. Insist on the patient's lying down when he has reached some place of shelter, and on thorough quiet at least for a time.

9. If you have persons to send for medical aid and appliances, make use of them at once; but remember that your directions and messages cannot possibly be too clear, too short, or too simple. A written message is of far more value than one sent by word of mouth, especially to the surgeon.

10. Have no useless talking to or in the hearing of the sufferer; and when he is fairly housed, banish from his room without mercy all except those necessary for his comfort and attendance;

let these, too, be as few in number as the circumstances will allow.

In all cases of other than very slight injuries, surgical aid should be procured as speedily as possible. The directions in this little book are by no means intended to supersede the resorting to educated skill. They may form a convenient code of rules to be acted on until the surgeon shall arrive; or if due professional aid cannot be obtained, then the injury must continue to be treated on the principles here sketched out.

CHAPTER I.

§ 1.—*Articles requisite for Immediate Dressings.*

THE articles necessary for the immediate dressing of wounds are not very numerous, nor are they, under ordinary conditions, difficult to meet with.

1. *Water* will be necessary,—most frequently it will be needed almost, if not quite, cold; or, if more grateful to the patient, it may be used lukewarm.

2. *Sponges* are a very great convenience; they should not be so large as to be unwieldy nor should they be loose in fibre, but rather small in size, of close texture, yet perfectly soft. All extraneous matter should have been washed out of them—such as bits of sea-sand, shells, &c.,—and the sponges should be well scalded with

boiling water before they are used. If the sponges have been used for cleansing unhealthy sores or for the application of medicated lotions, it is far the best that they should be destroyed when their use is at an end. There are many cases on record where it would seem that sponges have conveyed noxious matters from one patient to another.

3. *Flannel* will be the best material to use for the cleaning of a wound in the absence of sponge: it should not have been used for other purposes.

4. *Lint* is the material of its kind best adapted for surgical purposes. If it be not at hand, *soft cambric* or *lawn, e.g.*, a well-worn pocket-handkerchief, may be used in its place.

5. *Oil-silk, thin gutta-percha tissue,* or *oiled paper,* have their uses in keeping moist pieces of lint, linen, &c., which may have been wetted with water and applied to the injured part; the tissue being cut in

all its measurements a little larger than the piece of lint upon which it is placed.

6. *Plasters.* These exist in great variety of form: of all the ordinary adhesive plasters diachylon plaster is the most useful; though isinglass and court plasters have their advantages. The indications and the mode of applying plasters will be noted further on: it will be sufficient here to note that they are used in strips more or less broad, but the narrower the better, and long according to exigency; and that the adhesive material should be thoroughly softened by exposure to steam of boiling water or to a fire before the strip is applied. A convenient mode of softening plaster, is to pour into a basin, cup, or tin some boiling water; then to the outside of this vessel apply the reverse side of the strip just before the attendant wishes to make use of it.

7. *Pieces of linen,* cravats, or pocket-handkerchiefs. These should be used only

when thoroughly clean, and will readily assume the form of pads or *compresses*—folded more or less compactly and into shape as the case may require, they may be applied upon or at the side of wounded parts. As *bandages* or *supports* they may be used to encircle a limb, to retain dressings upon it, &c., and may be systematically described as used in form of the oblong, or square, the triangle, the cravat, and the cord. These titles sufficiently describe the various purposes to which they may be applied, and the requisite mode of folding. Two or three ordinary full-sized pocket-handkerchiefs will be sufficient for the immediate dressing of most injuries. Lastly, in the form of *slings* similar pieces of stuff may be employed to support an injured arm or hand.

The material whether silk, cotton, or linen is of secondary importance; and, therefore, if cravats or pocket-handkerchiefs be not at hand in sufficient number, strips or pieces of the proper size may be obtained from almost any part of the underclothing now worn by either sex.

8. *Splints* are specially needed in cases of fracture. They should be of tolerably firm material, adapted in a measure to the shape and contour of the injured limb, and may be fastened on, at all events for a time, by the cravat-bandages just named. It is best as a rule that they should be made of pieces of *wood* cut by a saw to the required width and length, and of such thickness as to afford support without being unnecessarily cumbrous and heavy. In the absence of wood, very efficient splints may be made of wheat-straw cut to the required length and taken up in such quantity that the due strength is obtained. Pieces of bark will answer admirably. If the accident has happened near to a house there will be little trouble in procuring some pieces of pasteboard, a hat, or a bonnet-box which may be sacrificed for the required end. Metal may occasionally be found in the shape required,

e.g., zinc tube or spouting, which may be split with a knife into separate slips; these should be several in number, three or four inches in width, while the length must be regulated by the special circumstances of each case.

9. *Bandages or rollers* can hardly be spoken of as necessary in the very first treatment of local injuries; but if the treatment should remain in the hands of the non-professional from the impossibility of obtaining duly skilled advice, their employment will be found a very great convenience. They are merely strips of calico or linen of fairly strong make, of about three fingers' breadth, and in length from three to six yards. The latter length should not be exceeded, as the roll becomes inconveniently bulky for the hand.

The piece of material should first have been washed to get rid of the glaze and stiffening with which it is got up for sale —the selvage removed, and then the bandages torn off throughout their whole length from one piece so that there be no cross ridges from the joining of short lengths together. Then each bandage should be rolled up tightly and firmly on itself, the further end being held during the process or tied to some immovable object.

A roller should be put on a limb from its extremity upwards, no part being skipped or left uncovered by the bandage, or swelling of such part will very probably occur, and the roller too will become loosened and easily detached.

As limbs, too, are not uniform in bulk,

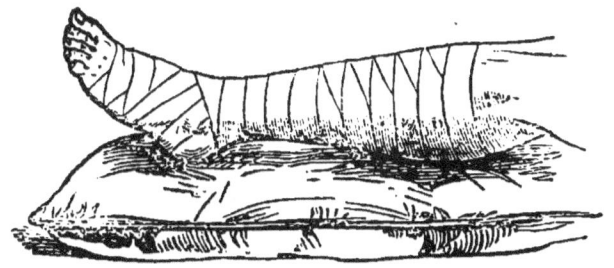

Fig. 1. Bandage on Leg and Foot.

but increase from below upwards, or from the terminal part to their junction with the trunk, so merely winding the roller round the limb will not answer—it must be put on *spirally;* each layer must cover over half of the preceding layer, and where sudden increase in bulk takes place, the roller must, once in each encircling of the limb, be turned half down upon itself, so that an accurate fitting may be secured. At the angles, formed by the joints, the figure of eight must be formed by the roller, the loops of this figure being applied, one round the limb above, the other below the joint; so leaving, in case of the knee and ankle, the kneepan and the heel respectively, without a covering of bandage.

It is impossible, in writing, to make thoroughly clear the mode of applying a roller—the knack, for such it is, can only be acquired by watching the process, and by frequently practising it either on some volunteer friend, or on a plaster model of a limb.

10. These details of necessary appliances

will have their fitting end by the naming a list of these articles, which might well be carried by travellers, couriers, and by some one out of a specified number of soldiers; the whole would form but a small package:—

        Lint.
        Compresses.
        Rollers.
        Sticking Plaster.
        Silk.
        Small Sponge.
        Tourniquet.
        Scissors.
        Tenaculum.
        Suture Needles.
        Lancet.
        Dressing Forceps.
        Scalpel.

The employment of some of these last-named agents will be referred to in future chapters.

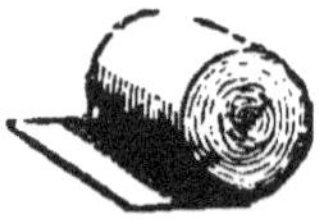

18   FIRST HELP IN ACCIDENTS.

Fig. 2. Roller.

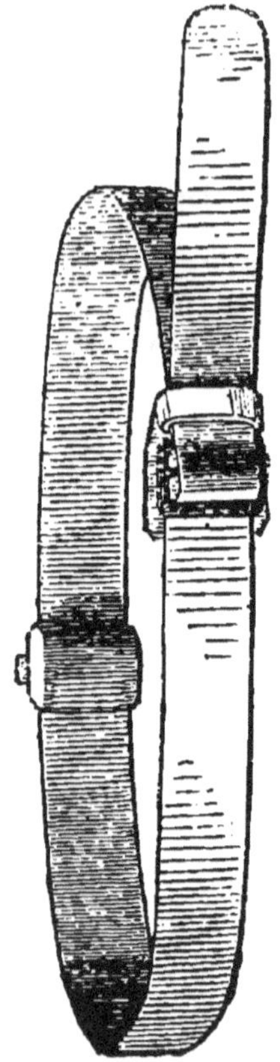

Fig. 3. Tourniquet.

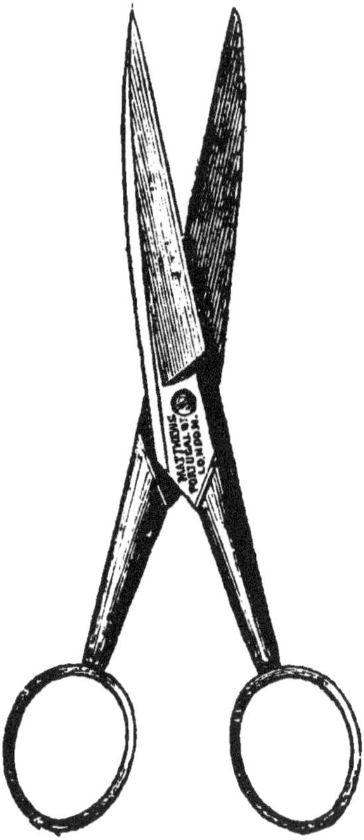

Fig. 4. Scissors.

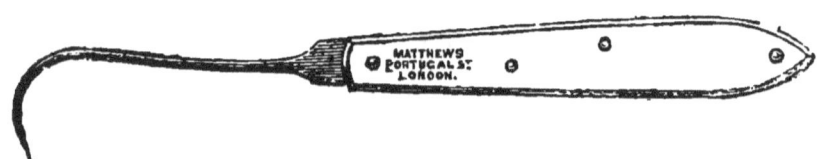

Fig. 5. Tenaculum.

ARTICLES FOR IMMEDIATE DRESSINGS.

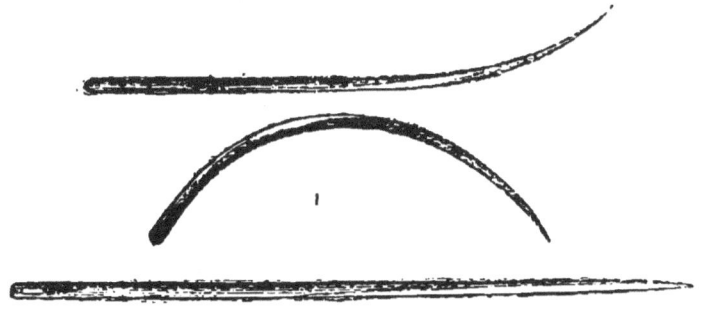

Fig. 6. Suture Needles.

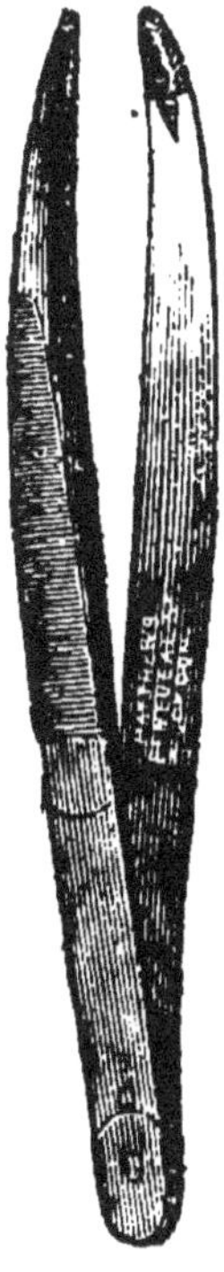

Fig. 7. Lancet.

Fig. 8. Dressing Forceps.

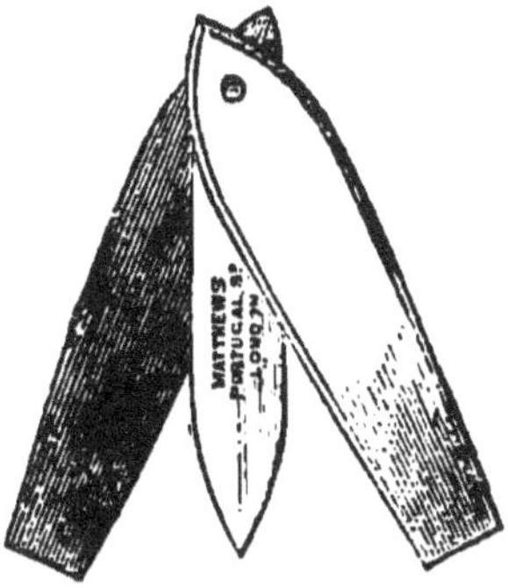

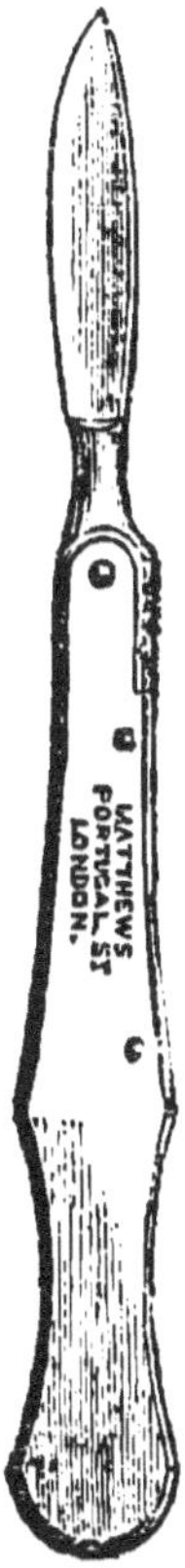

Fig. 9. Scalpel

§ 2.—*Subsequent Dressings: the local Applications of Cold and Heat. Leeches.*

This section may be at once declared to have reference to the secondary treatment of surgical cases in those instances where the coming of a qualified surgeon is long delayed, or where there is no chance of obtaining such skilled services. The forms in which the two great agents, cold and heat, can best be employed, will be here sketched: the cases in which one or the other must be resorted to, will be hereafter mentioned.

Increased heat in a part is one of the indications of inflammation having set in; and, for the purpose of diminishing this abnormal heat, *cold applications* are of much service. They may be used in form of—

1. *Evaporating Lotions.*—A single piece, one thickness, of linen should be dipped in the liquid, and laid on the injured part;

but no other covering is to be allowed over this. To secure evaporation, free access of external air is imperative, and the injured part should therefore be fully exposed, even though other parts of the same limb may need warm covering, flannel, &c. As the linen dries (and it may do so very rapidly), it must be wetted either by removing it and saturating it afresh with the lotion, or by filling a sponge with the lotion and squeezing it over the undisturbed linen covering. Cold water, reduced in temperature by dropping a piece of ice into the can, may be used in this mode; or medicated lotions, such as the following: two ounces of spirits of wine, or three ounces of brandy to a pint of cold water.

2. *Ice in Bladder or India-rubber Bag.*— Ice roughly pounded and put into a bladder, and this applied to the part, will furnish an intense degree of cold. In the use of this, the sensations of the patient should be consulted. Thus, if shivering and dis-

comfort follow upon the application of ice or other cold application, and this shivering be not merely a temporary but a lasting or recurring symptom, the cold should be discontinued. Should pain in and around the part come on, increased by each fresh supply of cold-producing material, this would furnish an immediate reason for change of dressing; and, lastly, change of colour to an intense paleness after a dark red, or even blue appearance, would demand the immediate though very gradual heightening of temperature in the application.

3. *Irrigation.*—This mode, as it is most easily regulated, will probably be found, after all, the most satisfactory. Place the patient on a bedstead with the damaged part exposed; beneath it stretch a piece of oilcloth, table-cover, or waterproof material, so arranged that water dripping on it shall be conducted off the bed into some convenient receptacle. Suspend from a part of the framework of a

venerable four-poster, from a stand purposely contrived, or from some hook placed in the ceiling, a can containing cold water—ice in this, if necessary—so that it shall hang almost directly over that part

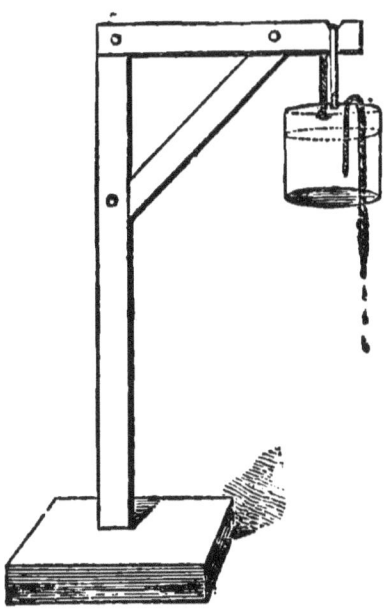

Fig. 10. Irrigation Stand.

to which cold is to be applied. The necessary continuous dripping may then be managed by hanging over the edge of the can a few threads of cotton, or a thin slip of lint, first well soaked; so that drop by drop the can may be emptied by capillary attraction, each drop falling on the part beneath. A special stand may be constructed for the purpose. The rapidity and force of the dripping will be well under control, and the exact point on which it falls can also be varied from time to time.

4. *Immersion.*—This will, as a rule, only be possible for some injury to one or other of the extremities, and but for a limited time.

Under certain conditions—such, for instance, as severe pain, collection of pus, &c., &c.—the *local application of heat* will prove of material advantage.

1. As *dry heat*, the application may be secured by the employment of small, well-stitched flannel bags, which have previously been filled with camomile-flowers, hops, with bran, or with sand. So filled, the bag should be heated by exposure to the fire, or by placing it in a well-warmed oven, and then applied to that part which may be the

seat of pain. When it is cooling, another bag, treated in the same way, should be substituted for the first one, and the required degree of heat should thus be kept up by a constant interchange.

2. As *moist heat*, in a minor degree, the use of *warm-water dressing* will answer the purpose. This will consist in the use of a double fold of lint or soft linen, well soaked in warm water, and applied to the part; while over this a covering of impermeable material, oiled silk, gutta-percha tissue, slightly larger than the lint, is carefully adapted.

3. *Moist heat to a greater amount* may be obtained by the employment of—

(a) *Fomentations.*—These are best managed by having some pieces of flannel or blanket, first cut to the required size, and thoroughly soaked in water, just so hot as to be grateful to the patient. The nurse's hand is no fair thermometer: what is pleasant to her case-hardened cuticle will often prove scalding to the patient. Place beneath the part to be fomented some waterproof or oilcloth, and then having had the flannels wrung nearly dry in a towel twisted by two people, wrap them round the limb, or apply them flat on the injured part, and then over the flannels some waterproof or thoroughly dry and thick covering, repeating the whole process as often as may be necessary.

(b) *Direct Immersion* may be practised when the foot or hand needs continuous application of heat, by placing the member in a shallow bath filled with water at the required temperature.

(c) *Poultices* may be made either of bread or of linseed meal; whichever material be employed, it should be so combined with boiling water as to form a soft, uniform, pulpy mass, free from lumps or foreign substances. So made, the mass should be spread, of moderate thickness, on linen or calico twice folded, and then applied to the part in pain. If linseed meal be preferred, as the more stimulating application of the two, or as more available for the purpose of hastening the process of suppuration, it is well to add a small quantity of hog's lard, so covering the whole surface of the poultice mass with a thin layer of melted fat.

Poultices should be changed more or less frequently, according to the special requirements of each case—never allowed to remain on the part affected after they have parted with the contained heat; for then they soon become cold, clammy, and unpleasant.

Mustard Plaster or Poultice is a ready and efficient mode of producing a temporary counter-irritation, and is frequently of much service. It is an application which can only be used to an unbroken surface of skin—the existence of superficial tear or abrasion of the cuticle forbids its employment. The mustard in fine powder should be mixed with boiling water to just such a consistence as if it were required for the dinner-table, and then the paste may at once be spread in moderate thickness either on a piece of leather, calico, or brown paper. On the face of the mustard, when spread, lay a piece of muslin or gauze, and let this be placed in close contact with the skin; by means of the muslin, the whole may be easily removed after from ten to twenty minutes' application, or such length of time as may be necessary to redden the skin thoroughly. The surface should then be well washed with a soft sponge, so as to get rid of any adherent fraction of the mustard.

As a subsequent dressing, a cambric handkerchief placed dry on the part, or, if it be preferred, moistened with oil or with some simple ointment, will give most relief; the smarting and redness pass off in a few hours.

Leeches are employed not unfrequently in the subsequent treatment of surgical cases, and so claim a passing mention. The indications for their use will be named in subsequent chapters. When it is deemed well to apply them, fresh leeches, or those which have not been recently in use, should certainly be chosen: the part to which they are to be applied cannot be too scrupulously cleaned, for the odour of perspiration, scents, &c., will prevent their taking hold; a small quantity of cream may be smeared lightly on the exact spot, and then the leeches applied, either *en masse*, by placing them in a wine-glass and inverting it over the part, or singly, so as to secure more accurate choice of situation. In the latter case, they may be applied by means of a leech-glass, or by taking them up one by one in the hand, covered with a towel, and so holding them to the point desired.

When fairly applied, leeches should be left to themselves: when gorged with blood, they will drop off. If it is desired to increase the loss of blood, warm fomentations may be employed and the flannels be removed frequently, or a bread poultice may be used in preference, changing it as it becomes cool. The arrest of bleeding from the bites will be secured usually without trouble, by the exposure of the part to the air by cold applications, or pressure with the finger. (For any further measures, see Chapter II.)

§ 3.—*Stimulants.*

Stimulants are agents of much value in the treatment of that condition of collapse and faintness which very commonly occurs after some physical injuries. The symptoms may be briefly sketched: The face is pale, bedewed with cold or clammy perspiration; the surface of body generally cold; the pulse flickering, perhaps hardly perceptible; the patient complains of the feeling of faintness, and may have nausea or even actual sickness; the breathing is sighing and irregular, and for a time there may be actual insensibility.

Now, under such conditions, there can be no question as to the propriety of inducing reaction by the administration of stimulants.

Coffee, given hot and strong, and in small quantity, is a safe and useful remedy.

Alcohol is more potent in its effects, and the good effect is produced more speedily. Brandy is the best spirit, given in more or less diluted form; failing this, rum or wine may be given. The best practical rule is to give a small quantity at first and watch its effect; if the surface becomes warmer, the breathing deeper and more regular, and the pulse at the wrist more perceptible, then there can be no question as to the advantage of giving even a little more; but if these signs of improvement are wanting,—if there be increase of insensibility and deepening of colour about the face with access of heat of skin, withhold alcohol entirely: it will but add to the mischief.

There can be no guide as to the quantity

necessary : the effect is the only indication. If much blood have been lost and the faintness be extreme, stimulants must be freely poured in, combining with their use thorough rest in the horizontal posture, and free access of air; but if there be no loss of blood, and nervous shock be alone the cause of the condition, the stimulant should be given cautiously, little by little, as it may seem advisable,—not in any single large dose.

When reaction, marked by return of colour to the face and warm perspiration, has once fairly set in, the use of any stimulant should be discontinued.

CHAPTER II.

BLEEDING:—WHERE IT MAY COME FROM, AND HOW TO ARREST IT.

§ 1.—*Blood Vessels.*

THE circulation of the blood throughout the body is carried on by the heart, as the central receiving and propelling organ, and by blood-vessels connected with it. Omitting all reference to the circulation through the lungs, arranged for the purpose of oxygenating and renewing that blood which has already supplied the general tissues; it will be well to speak of blood-vessels in the two divisions of *arteries* and *veins*, the former carrying bright red arterial blood to the different parts of the body from the heart, and having a distinct pulse at each beat of the heart; the latter carrying dull red or dark blood from the various parts of the frame back to the heart, and not possessing any distinct pulsation.

The main arteries pursue a tolerably direct course to the various limbs, and are placed, as a rule, not very near to the surface of the body; the position they occupy is the sheltered one on the inside of each limb.

The veins run in two sets—*superficial*, which are abundant in number, communicate freely with each other, and run a tortuous and twisted course—*deep*, which for the most part are side by side with the large artery, and are more direct.

An outline of the course of the main vessels will not be difficult to remember, and will be a necessary guide to the ready arrest of bleeding, be it more or less severe.

Notice.—In the following drawings, the *dark* vessels represent veins, and the *light* vessels arteries. The letter a in the drawings signifies *artery*, the v signifies *vein*.

BLOOD VESSELS.

1. Blood Vessels of the Head, Neck, and Upper Extremity.

There is on each side of the neck a large artery (carotid), which carries blood from the chest to the neck and head. It runs in a line from the inner end of the

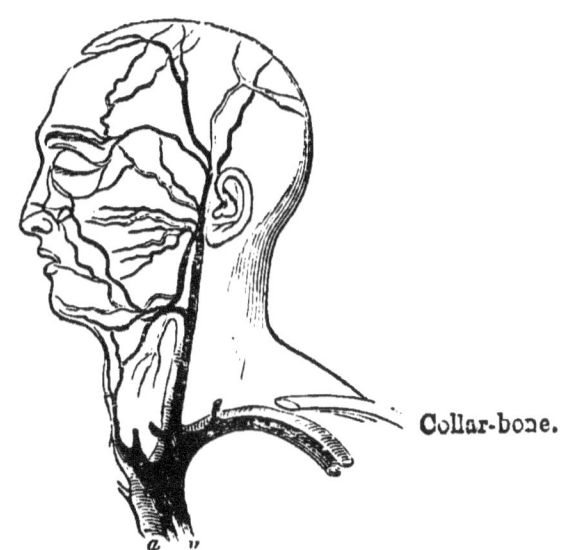

Fig. 11. Main Artery and Vein of the Neck and Head.

collar-bone to the angle of the lower jaw, and the pulsation is throughout fairly evident to the finger. The *deep* jugular vein lies very nearly parallel to the artery; the *superficial* jugular vein can readily be recognized under the skin.

To arrest bleeding in a wound of this artery, or one of its branches, pressure should be employed in a direction rather inwards and backwards, so as to press the vessel against the side-projections of the vertebral column.

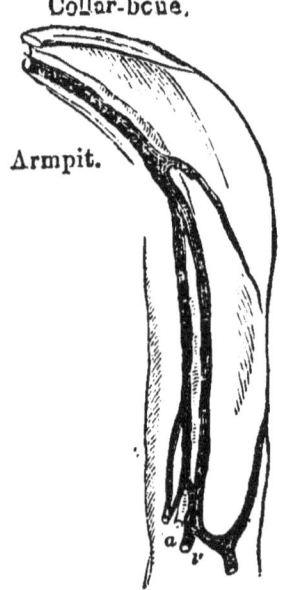

Fig. 12. Main Artery and Vein of Collar-bone, Armpit, and Upper Arm.

The great artery (subclavian) which supplies the upper extremity with blood, comes up out of the chest, and passes directly over the first rib in a direction outwards and downwards, towards the armpit. By pressing the thumb firmly into the neck, just behind the middle of the collar-bone, the pulsation may be detected; and in case of hæmorrhage from, in, or near the armpit, pressure should be kept up here for some time, either with a blunt piece of wood, with a rounded end, or with the handle of a common door-key wrapped in three or four folds of linen. The pressure will diminish or entirely prevent the blood current by the mechanical flattening of the vessel against the first rib. In the armpit it is not difficult to feel the artery (axillary) beating, by pressing the thumb or finger deeply towards the apex of the hollow, and pressure may be made by fixing the vessel between the fingers and the arm-bone at its upper part.

From this point the artery (brachial) runs onwards to the elbow, keeping always to the inside of the arm, and on the inner side of the prominent muscle of the upper arm. It is accompanied by parallel veins; throughout its course the artery is easily controlled by properly applied pressure, and, indeed, it is well for the reader to remember, that in wounds of the fore-arm or hand, accompanied by excessive arterial bleeding, the loss of blood may most satisfactorily be arrested by compressing this artery about the middle or lower third of its course.

Just below the bend of the arm, the main artery divides into two large branches—one (radial) taking the line of the outer bone, the other (ulnar) lying almost parallel with the inner bone. Both are in the greater part of their course rather deeply situated, and well covered by muscles, so that the detection of their pulsation is far from easy. At the wrist-joint both vessels may be felt beating, and to them in this situation pressure can well be applied.

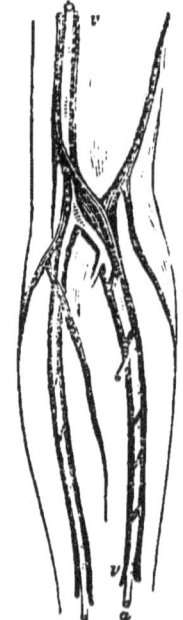

Fig. 13. Main Artery and Vein of Elbow and Fore Arm.

Certain branches pass onwards to the hand, forming arches more or less well marked, and from these, again, the fingers are supplied by straight vessels. In the event of much bleeding from the hand, the checking it may be attempted by pressure on both vessels at the wrist: if this fails, compress the main artery on the inside of the upper arm.

The superficial veins of the upper extremity are sufficiently evident; those which occupy the flexure of the elbow should be attended to (fig. 13); in one of these it is usual for surgeons to perform *venesection;* but no person who has not had an anatomical education should venture on the operation in this place: there is danger of puncturing the brachial artery as it passes in front of the elbow-joint.

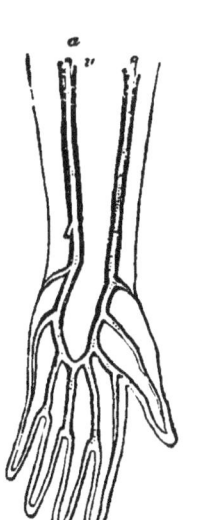

Fig. 14. Main Artery and Vein of Wrist-Joint and Hand.

The large arteries and veins within the cavities of the chest and abdomen, not being amenable to the simpler surgical measures, are here omitted.

2. *The Blood Vessels of the Lower Extremity.*

The large artery of the lower limb (femoral) passes downwards from the groin, lying about the middle of the crease of the groin, running almost at right angles to it. From this point of entrance, where its pulsation is very evident, and compression of it may be very easily managed, the vessel runs onwards, inclining to the inside, and ultimately turning half round the thigh-bone, so as to be felt quite behind it in the ham. In the upper three inches of its course

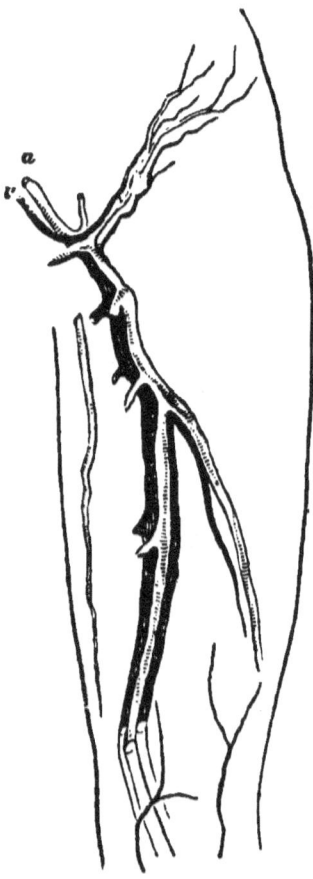

Fig. 15. Main Artery and Vein of Groin and Upper Leg.

the vessel can be felt with little difficulty; and if it should be wounded, compression at the point of injury, or at the line of entrance in the groin, will be effectual: the thumb is better in this instance than the handle of a door-key.

The large vein is internal to the artery at first, and then turns behind it.

If severe bleeding result on wound of the leg or foot, compression of the main vessel high up will be the most satisfactory plan.

As in the arm, so here, the main artery gives off two principal branches (anterior and posterior tibial) below the knee-joint; both

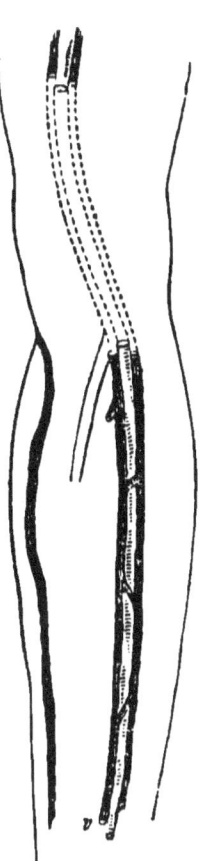

Fig. 16. Main Artery and Vein of Knee-Joint and Calves.

are deeply seated, and their pulsation, except near the ankle-joint, is not easily detected: one runs in front, the other behind the limb.

The foot is supplied by smaller branches from these two arteries.

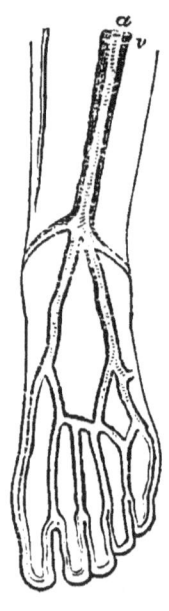

Fig. 17. Main Artery and Vein of Ankle and Foot.

The superficial veins are much larger than in the arm, and from wounds of them much bleeding may follow. The largest lies throughout on the inside of the limb, and is visible, if at all enlarged, throughout the whole length of its course.

A knowledge of the course of the principal blood-vessels may be obtained by a little practice in seeking out their course on the living subject— the pulsations will tell the line of the artery accompanied by its veins; the superficial veins will be evident from the deep colour of the blood seen through their thin walls.

§ 2.—*How to arrest Bleeding.*

From the descriptions already given, it will be manifest that bleeding may occur either from arteries or veins; and the first question to be settled in an instance of severe hæmorrhage should be, which kind of vessel has been injured.

A wounded artery will give out blood in separate jets, one closely succeeding another, and corresponding to the beats of the heart—*per saltum;* the blood, too, will be spirted out as florid, bright, red blood.

A vein, when wounded, will furnish dark red blood in a more or less continuous stream, but without the appearance of jet. If an artery deep down in the substance of a limb be wounded, the appearance of jet may be lost, and the blood, from retention in the deep wound, be darker, as it flows out, than bright arterial blood.

Wound of an artery may be treated—

1. *By Cold.*—This will only be applicable where the vessel or vessels are small and the jets minute; and the directing on the wound a stream of cold or iced water from a large sponge will promote the contraction of their walls and coagulation of the blood. The additional benefit of washing away all adhering clots will thus also be obtained. *Exposure to the air,* especially in the colder seasons, will have the same good result.

2. *By Pressure.*—This may be—

- (*a*) *Local;* applied to the bleeding point itself.

  The fingers form by far the best compressors. One or more should, after preparatory sluicing with cold water, be applied with moderate firmness to the exact point from which blood is found to issue, and there retained for some considerable time, pressing against bone or hard substance. As weariness will so be rapidly induced in the attendant's hand, a relay of assistants should be, if possible, provided, who may relieve one another in turn. This pressure should be kept up until the surgeon's arrival, if skilled aid can in any way be obtained.

Or after the thorough washing, *a graduated* compress may be applied to the wounded part. This is briefly a cone of soft material, such as lint, strips of linen, silk, &c., made up of numerous pieces, and so arranged that the apex of the cone shall be applied to the very bottom of the wound. One very small bit is first inserted, others one by one upon this, until a mass is applied sufficient to afford a resisting surface; and upon this, as a base, with the view of retaining the cone immovable, a piece of wood or a large coin may be firmly fixed by a cravat-bandage, or roller. The arrangements may be varied according to the exact locality of the injury and the means at hand; but as the final measure, a bandage applied over the whole limb, commencing at the terminal point and covering over the compress, will be of much service.

(b) *Distant* pressure may be employed, not of necessity to the wound itself, *e.g.*—

Finger pressure may be applied to the main artery of the limb, even several inches above the seat of injury, to prevent further access of hæmorrhage until skilled assistance can be got.

A *"vessel-compressor,"* or *"tourniquet,"* may be applied with much good, if the bleeding be anywhere below the middle of the thigh. (See p. 18, fig. 3.) It is hardly likely that in

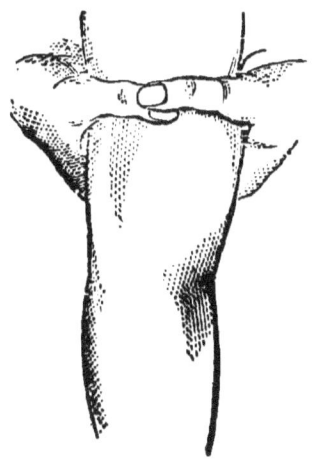

Fig. 18. Finger Pressure.

sudden emergencies the instrument specially made for the purpose will be at hand, but a substitute may be readily contrived thus:—
Tie tightly, at some little distance above the wound, a pocket-handkerchief or cravat once or twice passed round

the limb; then, obtaining a piece of tough stick, push it under the handkerchief, and, by turning the stick, twist the handkerchief more and more tightly, until the bleeding ceases.

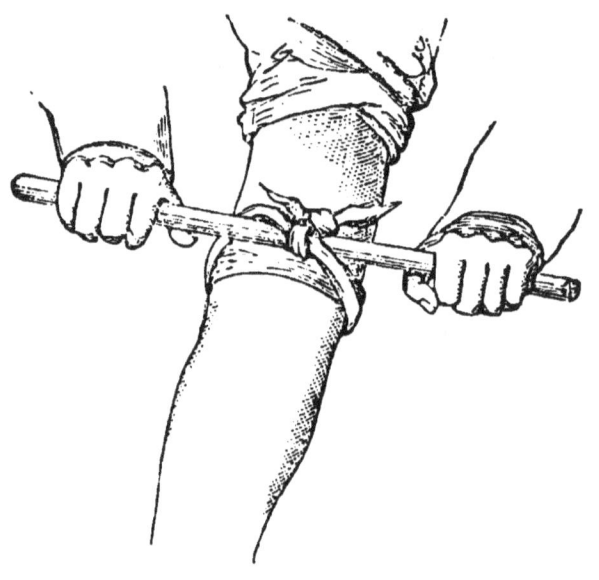

Fig. 19. Stick Tourniquet.

As soon as this result has been attained, fasten the stick by another handkerchief tied round stick and limb together. This rude tourniquet may save life not unfrequently, by enabling the injured person to be transported even for some distance, without fear of further bleeding.

3. *By Position.*—The cessation of bleeding is favoured and sometimes insured by merely raising the injured limb above the level; placing it, indeed, on an incline with hand or foot, as the case may be, much above the level of the trunk.

Forcible flexion of the knee and elbow joints will, too, in some persons effectually control bleeding occurring from a wound beyond these joints. The sides of the main vessel are approximated, and though the current of blood through its channel be not thoroughly stopped, yet both the size of the stream and its impetus are very much lessened. To carry out this purpose effectually, the arm should be forcibly bent at the elbow, and the fore arm and upper arm then bound together by a strong handkerchief tied tightly round them as high up as can well be managed. The leg should be so bent at the knee that the heel shall nearly or quite touch the buttock behind, and then the leg and thigh must be firmly bound together in this unnatural and not over-pleasant position.

4. *By the application of a Ligature.*—This simply implies the tying a piece of silk or thread tightly around the point from which blood is issuing. In most cases, some small artery is wholly or partially divided, and pressure and cold having failed to arrest the hæmorrhage, these further means may be resorted to. Only, be it understood, may this plan be employed if it be impossible to obtain surgical advice. These cases of uncontrollable bleeding call not unfrequently for further and more serious measures, which are not here named in detail, since they can only be carried out by skilled assistance.

If the cut be open, with widely separated edges, it will be possible sometimes at least to see the exact point from which blood issues. A common long stocking-needle, or, better still, a slightly curved or hook-shaped needle (called a tenaculum, see engraving on p. 18, fig. 5) may be plunged in for some little depth behind the bleeding point, and then brought out again through the tissues, so as to hold up on the needle-stem a fold of flesh or tissues, in which fold the point of bleeding may be detected.

The needle then must be held well forward, so as to tighten and bring the parts well into sight. Behind the needle a silken thread must be passed, and so tied that it shall embrace firmly the tissues held up, and so mechanically enclose within its grasp the divided point of the artery. The tenaculum may then be withdrawn; in a few days the silk will be loose from the textures ulcerating in the line of its constriction of them, and so may readily be drawn out. A fine packing-needle somewhat curved will be available in the absence of a tenaculum.

If a vein be wounded, and this the character of the blood-stream in tint and flow will mostly decide, pressure by finger or graduated compress will be most effectual.

The tourniquet is not to be used, nor is it advisable to employ a ligature to the bleeding point.

Excessive bleeding from leech-bites may be readily checked in this way—pass a common fine and straight sewing-needle through the tissues behind the bleeding point, and tie behind this tightly a piece of strong thread or silk. Remove both the needle and silk at the end of twelve hours.

CHAPTER III.

WOUNDS: THEIR VARIETIES AND TREATMENT.

THE mode of treatment of all wounds may be described as coming under four divisions:

1. By washing with sponge and warm or cold water, ensure the thorough removal of any material which may have been driven into the wound. Grains of sand, dirt, &c., should be got rid of by the use of water. Larger substances, fibre of linen, cloth, or clots of blood should be removed by the fingers or by surgical forceps (see p. 19, fig. 8)—the surface of the wound, in short, accurately cleaned.

2. Stop flow of blood, either by pressure, ligature, or position, as noted in Chapter II.

3. Bring the divided portions as nearly

as possible into contact, observing as guide for this purpose any mark on skin, natural fold or crease, &c., and when so adjusted retain them in their natural position:

(a) By plasters.—For this end the ordinary resinous adhesive plaster, court plaster, or isinglass plaster may be employed.

(b) By compresses and use of bandages.

(c) By stitches or sutures.—For this purpose needles of different shape and curve, and made so as to carry silk of sufficient strength, are employed (see p. 19, fig. 6); or common sewing-needles are available, with silk wound round them in the form of a figure of 8.

4. Favour the growing together of the divided edges by keeping the patient thoroughly at rest, feeding him lightly, and keeping the functions of the body in proper order.

WOUNDS.

Incised Wounds or Cuts.

These are made with clean cutting instruments, in everyday life by razor, knife, glass, &c.; in military engagements by blows with sword or sabre.

After cleansing the lips of the wound thoroughly from all extraneous substances, and checking the bleeding, the two edges should be fitted together as closely as possible. If the wound be on the head, the hair on each side may be tied across the wound at short intervals, so as to keep the edges in contact.

If plasters are used, they should be applied in strips of length and breadth proportionate to the injury inflicted. Having first softened the plaster surface, one end of the strip should be closely applied to the sound skin, at right angles to the cut, and at some distance from its edge; then the wound being closed by temporarily holding together by the fingers, carry the strip across the line of contact, and affix it to the sound skin at a like distance on the other side of the cut. Each strip so applied should lie parallel with the preceding ones, and when a sufficient number have been put on, a compress of three or four folds of linen, placed over and in the line of the wound, should be applied, and a few turns of a roller over all will keep this in place.

In removing or changing plasters, the ends should first be raised, and both lifted up from the outside to the centre, so that no dragging may take place at the injured part. If fresh plasters are needed, apply the strips one by one as the old ones are removed, not exposing the wound to the risk of gaping for want of support.

Should the wound be deep or extensive, it will be well to employ sutures—these may be of silk, thus applied:—

A needle threaded with silk is passed through the skin and tissues just beneath, on one side of the wound *from without inwards*, and then through a corresponding point of the other lip *from within outwards*. The silk so carried through must be tied in a firm knot. The separate stitches should be from half an inch to an inch apart.

The silk may remain undisturbed for three or four days, and if then cut through on one side of the knot, the stitch may be easily taken out.

Or a common sewing needle may be used thus, forming what is called "*the twisted suture.*" Having introduced it at first as if it were a needle carrying silk, the needle is allowed to remain holding both lips of the wound in contact; and over this needle a piece of silk may be twisted, so as to form the figure of 8, and to embrace with its loops the two projecting ends of the needle, thus holding more thoroughly even than on the other plan the divided edges in close contact. After three days the needle may be drawn out, and the silk will then fall off.

Much may be done by position only, in keeping the edges of an incision close together, especially in wounds of the hand or arm: thus a wound on the inner or front surface of the arm will need bending of the elbow; on the back surface, extension of the arm.

If plasters, &c., be not in readiness, some support may be given to the divided edges by wrapping strips of linen moistened with cold water round the part injured; these will adhere more or less closely, and may either be allowed to remain or be removed to allow the use of a more accurate kind of dressing.

It may be well here to say, that even though thorough division of a part may have taken place (*e.g.*, a finger or a toe, or even though a portion of the nose or ear may have been completely severed), still an attempt to re-unite the divided parts ought to be made, and success will very frequently follow the attempt.

The directions given above will, in the majority of instances, tend to the cure of an incised wound by—

The immediate or primary process: that of rapid adhesion between the surfaces which have been divided, but are within a short time closely brought together and retained in absolute contact. If this desirable result be attained, there will be no appearance of discharge of matter or watery fluid—the part will not become the seat of pain—especially the feeling of distension from within will not be complained of; and, as time passes on, the smarting of the wound will more and more subside: then for a day or two at least the dressings may be undisturbed, and when removed (and this should be done only by degrees) a certain support should be afforded to the injured part by a repetition, in some modified degree, of the same plan of dressing.

The incised wounds with which soldiers may have to deal in assisting their wounded comrades will be those inflicted with the sword; their immediate dressing will best be confined to the arrest of bleeding by pressure, *direct* on the wound itself or *remote* on the main vessel of the limb (see Chapter II.)—to the maintaining, so far as may be done, the position best suited to fulfil the necessities of each special injury, and to the retaining by cravat or roller simple dressings or compresses upon the wound.

The transporting the sufferer to the hospital will be imperative—on the ready attention of a skilled hand the result of a severe incised wound will very much depend. The motionless condition of the injured part and the easy removal of the whole body are points also to be borne in mind.

But this rapid cure of incised wounds

cannot always be obtained. It may be said, in passing, that of this kind of repair, these clean cut wounds are alone capable; in other cases, the injury will be repaired in a different mode, *i.e.*, by—

The secondary modelling or moulding process.—Here the surfaces of the wound which have failed to unite by primary adhesion are found to be covered with minute conical elevations, called granulations, and these are bathed in matter which is yellowish-opaque, and of the consistence of cream; to this the term of "pus" is applied. Even at this stage, if the opportunity be watched, it is not unfrequently possible to procure a growing together of two surfaces so covered, the granulations fitting into, so to speak, and inosculating with each other More frequently, however, the wound is healed by gradually filling up to the level of surrounding parts by the steady multiplication of these granulations, one above another, until the gap is fairly obliterated.

Therefore, supposing an incised wound to be the seat of throbbing pain, the pain of a distension from within, and the edges to have become red and inflamed, or pale and flabby-looking, the closely applied dressings should be removed, the retained pus allowed to escape, a few strips of plaster be applied to keep the divided parts near to, if not in absolute contact with each other, and the whole wound dressed with water-dressing or bread poultice, &c. The exact application, whether of cold or heat, may be safely left to the liking and feelings of the patient, but it should be continued so long as the discharge of matter lasts, and until there is formation of new skin and sound healing of the external wound.

The new flesh may rise above the level, be unnecessarily exuberant, and so retard healing; if this be the case, a piece of blue stone (sulphate of copper) may be lightly rubbed over the whole, or some pressure used with a piece of dry lint for a day or two.

Punctured Wounds or Pricks.

The most serious injuries coming under this head will be bayonet wounds received in battle. As soon as possible, soldiers meeting with such injuries should be transferred to the hospital. An early treatment at the hands of a comrade should be devoted to arrest of hæmorrhage by local pressure (fingers or bandage), and to the preserving during transport perfect immobility of the part injured.

In civil practice, punctured wounds apparently very trivial are yet sometimes most serious in their results. The entrance of a thorn deeply into the tissues has again and again given rise to much irritative fever, deep collections of matter, and even to most serious illness.

The rules of treatment should be to extract the foreign body, if it be possible, with tweezers or with the point of a needle, and this extraction will often be aided by a free division of the skin and deeper tissues by a lancet or knife. Then the application of moisture, as a large bread poultice, will give much relief, and the arm or leg should be kept thoroughly at rest.

If inflammation should follow, with throbbing pain, lines of redness running from the injured point to the trunk, and general fever, the non-professional (if other advice be impossible) will give most relief by applying leeches in good number near the seat of injury, and then abundance of warmth and moisture. If pain continue, and swelling of the part come on, an incision with a lancet, so made that the surgeon's cut shall include the line of the original wound, will often give vent to contained matter and so afford great relief. After this, the wound may be expected to heal slowly by the process of filling up by granulations.

Lacerated or Torn Wounds.

These wounds do not entail the same risk of severe bleeding as incised or punctured injuries: and the soldier dealing with them, as caused for the most part by missiles discharged from guns, or by stones, pebbles, &c., thrown up by cannon shot, will have to attend to—

The removal of foreign substances from the surface of the wound, the application of cold-water dressings, and the easy and quick removal of the sufferer.

In civil practice, the simplest form of this kind of injury, only a *scratch,* is yet, if it be irritated by dirt, by movement of the limb, or by violent exertion, very often followed by awkward consequences. Inflammation may spread from the finger up the arm, and matter form deeply near the wound. The same treatment noted in punctured wounds, leeches, heat, with incisions to let out matter, must here also be resorted to.

It may be well to add, that although some kind of support, as by a few strips of plaster or a compress, &c., may be of service, no close apposition should be attempted. The edges are not likely, from the irregular character of the wounds, and from the force employed in their infliction, to grow together. The cure by granulation should be aided by rest, warmth, and position.

In the less severely lacerated wounds, it may often be well to try to procure *healing under a crust or scab.* Thus the wound may be treated by the early application of a piece of lint soaked in blood or in Friar's balsam, and this artificial coating may remain undisturbed, even for many days.

If much pain and feeling of distension supervene, the covering may be raised at one part only; but if there be much discharge, it will be requisite to take it entirely away, and dress the granulating sore with water dressing, poultice, &c.

Contused Wounds.

These are wounds made by the falling on the part of some heavy blunt-edged material. The weight of the object and the force of its fall bruise and crush the edges of the cut, and no bringing together will induce them to unite with each other. Before the breach of surface can be repaired, the damaged part must separate as a slough or piece of dead tissue, and then the wound may become clean, secrete healthy pus, and heal by granulations.

Cold or warm applications may be employed at first, and poultices or water-dressing will complete the repair.

Gunshot Wounds.

Bleeding in these injuries is not very frequently found to occur immediately.

Simple water-dressing, retention of such dressings by roller or cravat, and removal as speedily as possible to the regimental surgeon, are the means to which the soldier may well resort.

One of the immediate consequences is *shock*, more or less severe; death even may take place very speedily from this one cause. Some stimulant should be soon given, and the head kept low. Encouragement by voice or gesture is always advisable.

These cases only can be treated by a non-professional when the shot has injured some part not material to life, or where it has passed through a limb without damage to the bone or the large blood-vessels. The external wound may, as in the instance of the face, &c., be brought together with strips of plaster, and dressings be applied on the general principles already sketched, while perfect rest must be maintained, and the patient must be lightly fed.

The remarks hitherto made in treating

of wounds have had reference for the most part to their primary or immediate treatment. But it may well happen that medical assistance is not to be had, and after some short time a wound, be it incised or lacerated, will need further attention. This should be remembered as a cardinal rule, that any union obtained by the use of sutures or plasters, position, &c., although it may be but slight compared with the whole extent of the injury, should not be lightly disturbed. Great gentleness will therefore be necessary in after dressings. First, the plasters, compresses, &c., very possibly partially at least adherent to the wound, and matted with blood or puriform discharge, should be well soaked with warm water, and when so softened, are then to be removed. The surface of the wound should be gently cleansed with sponge and water, and clean dressings applied.

These may be, if the edges are red and

angry looking, with but scanty secretion of matter, still softening and moist, such as poultices and water-dressing. If the wound look healthy, and the pus discharged be satisfactory, the water-dressing will still be available, and later on some astringent or drying applications will be advisable. Hardly any sore will pass through all its stages to perfect recovery without deriving some benefit from an occasional change of application. The best local astringents are perhaps such as—

Zinc Lotion, thus made :—
> Sulphate of zinc, 20 grains.
> Water, half a pint.

It may be used with lint; the lint well saturated with the lotion and then applied.

Calamine Ointment :—
> One part of yellow bees' wax.
> Two parts of sweet (olive) oil or lard.

These melted together and well mixed,

not, however, allowed to boil; and as the mass is cooling, one part of calamine powder may be stirred in.

As deodorizing agents, to counteract fœtid discharges, &c., a solution of permanganate of potash (Condy's patent fluid), used in the proportion of a teaspoonful to a pint of water, will be of service. This may be used as a lotion to the wound, and also placed about the room in saucers, plates, &c.

The chlorides of lime and soda, or the chloride of zinc, diluted with water in due proportion as their vendors direct, may be employed with advantage.

CHAPTER IV.

BRUISES AND CONTUSIONS.

THESE will vary from a slight condition of local injury to a very severe crushing. They result either upon a fall from some height, or are caused by a weight falling upon some part of the body. The local changes are not to be mistaken. There will not be wound of the skin, but swelling appears within a greater or less time, with dark blue discoloration; the latter depending on the rupture of small vessels beneath the skin by the force of the blow. The swelling may be even very great, and the distension of the skin will so give rise to much pain.

The two necessary points of treatment are to afford moisture to the part bruised, and to insist on thorough rest. It will usually be most grateful to the patient to have warm applications, a large bread poultice, or hot fomentations, by frequently renewed flannels; these soften the skin and relieve the pain. But in some cases cold water is most refreshing. A lotion of arnica may be employed—

> Tincture of arnica, 1 part.
> Water, from 5 to 8 parts.

This, by some surgeons, is thought to be of much good in relieving pain, and also in promoting the absorption of the blood poured out.

It may be that the pain continues in spite of these means, and if so, the application of leeches in good number, twenty to thirty if a limb be much injured, may give much relief. The subsequent bleeding may be increased and encouraged by the employment of large bread poultices or hot flannels.

For some days the patient must keep quite at rest. The change of colour in the injured part from black, through many varieties of shades, to a dingy yellow, is due to alteration in the effused blood, and should be looked on as a necessary condition, and also as an indication of slow recovery.

These rules of treatment will only apply to the less severe instances of contusion. Where the weight has been very great, and the resulting injury very severe, it is not possible that it can be dealt with satisfactorily, except by medical knowledge. All that can be done is to support the injured part, especially during removal. Apply cold-water dressing and cravat bandage, obtaining the requisite help as soon as possible.

CHAPTER V

BURNS AND SCALDS.

THESE injuries, the consequence respectively of contact of fire and boiling compounds, with the structures of the human frame, have so much of similarity in their appearance and in the treatment required, that they may be mentioned here under the same head.

Three different degrees of burning or scalding have been accepted by systematic writers:—

1. When the contact has been but for a very short time, and the injury is that of redness and inflammation of the skin with coincident severe pain.

2. Where blisters have formed, from a greater amount of heat being applied.

3. When there is destruction of skin and the underlying structures, they are changed into a yellow or black mass, and all vitality is destroyed; the damaged parts separate as sloughs, leaving large gaps to be filled up by granulation.

The amount of pain will vary much in different cases. On the whole, its presence, if it be not of unbearable severity, is rather of good omen than otherwise; the absence of suffering must be taken in extensive burns and scalds to indicate extreme and imminent danger.

Much of the probable result will depend on the part injured, and the extent of surface which has been implicated. Thus severe burns about the chest and abdomen, particularly in children, are almost always fatal; those, too, of the lower extremities are more dangerous than the same injuries affecting the face, neck, and arms.

The Treatment of Burns.

First put out the blaze, if the clothes have caught fire. Do not on any account let the sufferer run about—every draught of air will fan the flame; but throw him at once on the floor, and wrap him up in folds of carpet, hearth-rug, curtains, table-cloths, &c.; or if the person can only think of the plan, he may well roll himself over and over on the floor until the flames are mechanically put out. Then let the patient be taken to bed, and if there be much shock to the system, with faintness or prostration, some hot coffee or stimulants should at once be given.

Next remove the clothes, cutting them away from any injured part. If the skin should adhere to some part of the under dress, cut the dress, but be careful not to tear through or injure the skin where blisters have formed.

The keeping the air away is the main

point to be looked to in the dressing, and this end may be attained by using—

Dry applications—such as flour liberally shaken on from a common flour-dredger, or finely-powdered starch, cotton-wool, or wadding in sheets, as used for ladies' dresses, only taking care to use the covering so freely that the air shall be well excluded.

Moist applications are best used warm—more grateful to the patient than if they are applied perfectly cold.

The carron oil—a mixture of lime-water and oil in equal parts—may be freely used, and over this layers of cotton wool; or the parts may be brushed with turpentine and then covered with a mixture of equal parts of turpentine and resin ointment spread on linen or wadding.

Again, the part may be first painted over with oil, and on this surface flour be dredged. It will adhere more closely than if flour alone be used. Scraped potatoes are easily obtained also.

The use of applications which are warm and stimulating is to be preferred to the employment of cold and simply soothing compounds. The first dressings should remain undisturbed at least for twenty-four hours or longer, and then be repeated in the same or in a modified form; the subsequent treatment may be by using calamine ointment, water-dressing, or poultices; but so many casualties are attendant upon the after treatment of severe burns, that medical aid should be obtained without any delay. Where much surface skin is destroyed, death may occur from congestion or inflammation of internal organs, or from effusion within the cavity of the skull. At a later period, death most frequently follows from the wearing out of physical strength, by the long continuance of exhausting discharges, &c.

It will be well to name, that in the event of lime getting on the front of the eye or under the eyelids, water should *not* be employed. Washing with vinegar will neutralize the caustic properties of the lime, and any fractional bits may afterwards be removed by the use of a feather lightly applied, by a camel-hair pencil lightly used, or by a fold of linen screwed to a point. Acute inflammation of the eye must be looked for after such an accident, and though even with immediate medical aid the organ may be much damaged, without it sight will be almost certainly sacrificed.

The local application of leeches around the lids, and frequent use of warm fomentations, constitute all that can be safely done by non-professional hands.

Chemical agents sometimes come in contact with the skin.

Acids.—As oil of vitriol, aquafortis, &c.; an alkaline solution should at once be applied—carbonate of soda or magnesia dissolved in water; in the absence of these remedies, common soap made into a thick lather with soft water; olive oil may afterwards be used freely, and the ulcers which may remain must be treated on general principles.

Alkalies — as quicklime, caustic ammonia, or potash—need the opposite treatment; weak vinegar or much-diluted acids should be at once applied.

Corrosive sublimate is rendered inert by the free use of white of egg. *Butter of antimony,* by applying water in abundance. *Nitrate of silver,* unless very freely employed, will not do much local mischief. Salt and water will decompose this silver salt.

CHAPTER VI.

EFFECTS OF COLD, FROZEN LIMBS, ETC.—
EFFECTS OF HEAT.—SUNSTROKE.

§ 1.—*Cold, Exposure to, the Effects of.*

WHEN cold is severe, and there has been long-continued exposure to its influence, the effects on the human body are distinctive and well marked. The cooling of the external surface is accompanied by internal congestion of the principal organs; the skin becomes pale, the muscles stiffened, and the circulation in the external parts is much lessened. The nervous system then is affected: the sufferer will complain of giddiness and inability to guide himself, and then of extreme weariness and desire to sleep. If this wish be indulged, complete stupor and death will only too certainly follow.

All these symptoms approach with far greater rapidity in those who have their nervous energies depressed by intoxication, or by long-continued exertions which have induced exhaustion. Insufficient supply of food will also materially influence the injurious effects of severe cold.

If the cold be very severe, freezing and absolute death of some portion of the frame may occur. If any considerable extent be frozen, it is very unlikely that the vitality of the part can be recovered.

Local injury may, however, thus happen and be repaired. The nose, ears, face, or extremities may suffer—the part first becomes dull, bluish red in colour, the power of moving it is soon lost, and sensation then disappears; the natural colour is changed, and the damaged portion is thoroughly pale, shrivelled, and tallowy-looking.

When the general effects of cold are

manifested on the system as a whole, by insensibility and torpor, the treatment must commence :—

1. By subjecting the body to a temperature only a few degrees above the freezing point. This may be done in some convenient room without a fire, or in the open air.

2. The clothes should be cautiously removed, and friction commenced with snow over the trunk and parts which have suffered most. The rubbing is the material agent for good: this may be continued after a short time by flannels.

3. The body may be placed in a bath of cold water if snow be not at hand, and friction even there still kept up. By the addition of water, a little warmer each time, the temperature of the surface may be increased.

4. If there be return of surface warmth, or an attempt at respiration occur, the body should at once be removed from the

bath, or the snow covering taken away, and the surface then wiped thoroughly dry.

5. Artificial respiration may be set up, according to the directions given in Chapter XI.

6. The bed in which the patient is placed should, in the first place, be cold, and the temperature of the room may be raised by degrees until it reaches a fairly genial warmth. Some nourishment should be given so soon as the patient can swallow; warm milk, broth, a little warm wine and water, &c.

If local effects only have resulted from the exposure to cold, the part affected should be covered with snow and well rubbed, or a bath of very cold water may be employed until the power of movement and sensation in slight measure return. When this point of recovery has once been reached, friction with flannels continued for some time will be of most advantage.

The change from cold to heat must not

be too sudden, or mortification, local death of the part which has been injured, will certainly follow. The part will then have lost its vitality and must separate. But this process, especially if it involves much of the surface or the whole circumference of a limb, will entail great risk to life, and can only be treated by qualified medical skill.

An amount of protection against the local influence of severe cold may be obtained by rubbing the exposed parts with fat or tallow, so as to give them a thorough coating. It has also been suggested to employ the finest carpenter's mouth glue, made into a thick paste with cold water, and to use this spread on linen, as a local covering for the defence against external cold.

§ 2.—*Influence of Heat—Sunstroke, &c.*

The general effects of the opposite condition, extreme heat, deserve notice. In

EFFECTS OF HEAT.

another place (Chapter V.) the local effects are treated under the heading of Burns and Scalds.

When there is exposure to the rays of a hot sun, as in India, for example, especially if the head be not properly protected, the conditions of heat,—apoplexy, coup-de-soleil, or sunstroke, speedily show themselves. Even in England, during some of the hot days of summer, cases of the same kind have happened. More especially may these symptoms be expected to occur in those who are depressed from much physical exertion, or from defective or improper supply of food. So soldiers on a march under a vertical sun, carrying heavy knapsacks, accoutrements, &c., are the most frequent sufferers. Indulgence in alcoholic liquors certainly increases the tendency to the affection.

The man most probably first becomes faint and giddy, turns pale, and may fall down insensible. As the symptoms advance there is flushing of the face, with increased action of the heart and laboured breathing, and then thorough coma, upon which in a few hours death will supervene. Slighter symptoms may occur, and either pass away under judicious treatment, or slowly merge into the severer form.

Treatment.

The patient should be removed into a cool place if possible, or, at least, some shade should be procured so as to ward off the intense heat.

The head should be kept cool with wet cloths, only applied of thin material and in a single layer, so that constant evaporation may go on from the wetted surface, so keeping the head thoroughly cool.

It is neither necessary nor advisable that bleeding should be resorted to without positive proof of its necessity. This doubtful point can only be decided by medical authority; and, in the absence of qualified assistance, the lancet should certainly not be used.

As the affection appears, from the testimony of well-skilled observers, to depend on shock to the nervous system and depression of nervous energy, so those remedial measures are best which rouse the exhausted tissues to fresh action and supply support to them. Hence, so soon as the patient can swallow, stimulants, wine, brandy and water, &c., with nourishing food should be given.

Many more recoveries are noted under this plan of treatment than when blood has been abstracted, and means employed which tend to diminish more or less directly general nerve-power.

CHAPTER VII.

SPRAINS—DISLOCATIONS.

A *DISLOCATION* is, as its name implies, a slipping out of place. One bone is separated by violence from its attachment to its fellow; is tilted out of the socket which it properly occupies, and is then said to be dislocated. This injury is accompanied by more or less stretching and tearing of the tough fibrous textures which keep bones in their proper position.

A *Sprain* may be defined as a dislocation begun but not completed; that is, the bones entering into the formation of a joint are violently separated, the ligaments torn or much stretched, but there is no actual persistent displacement of the surfaces of the respective bones

To speak of *sprains* first. The joints in which these injuries most frequently happen are the wrist and ankle; they are usually consequent upon some sudden and unnatural movement of the joint, followed by aching pain and more or less swelling; but the bony points and their relations one to another will be, on comparing the injured with the uninjured joint, found to be precisely the same. Sprains must be treated by thorough rest. If the wrist be injured, a sling must be constantly worn; if the ankle, the patient must lie or sit with his leg lying flat and immovable on a couch or stool.

The immediate and continuous application of cold, by the employment of irrigation (see Chapter I.), will prevent much effusion into the injured joint, and also bar the occurrence of acute inflammation. This should be kept up more or less regularly for some two or three days, and then a bandage, wet with cold water, may be closely applied. When pain has quite subsided, and the sprained joint is simply weak, much good may be obtained by casing it with strips of soap plaster, each one as it is put on slightly overlapping the preceding one, so as to limit the range of movement, and afford an efficient and continual support.

If there should be much pain, and this be not relieved by cold and rest, the application of leeches, ten to twenty, will very probably give relief. Let their removal be followed by a large warm bread poultice, so as to encourage the bleeding.

But at the outset, the sufferer from a sprained wrist or ankle should be reminded that the injury will be very slow in passing quite away. The joint will remain weak, slightly swollen, and in some pain, it may be, even for a long time, in spite of all remedial measures. Surgical experience thoroughly confirms, in this case, the popular dictum, "that a bad sprain is worse than a broken bone."

Dislocations.—These injuries can be recognised by three principal symptoms :—

Deformity.—An alteration in shape as compared with the opposite side of the body. The limb affected will be altered in length, it may be shorter or longer than in its natural state.

Loss of usual movements of the joint.—A bystander may seize the limb and move it at the cost of some pain to the patient, though this even will be in limited area; but the sufferer himself will be found on inquiry to have the power of performing some only of the ordinary movements. The arm, if the shoulder be dislocated, cannot be raised upwards, as before.

Absence of signs which indicate a fracture.—There will be no alteration in the appearance of the shaft of a bone, no crackling, grating, or rubbing of the fractured ends, surgically called crepitus. Absence, also, of an excessive and abnormal mobility at the injured part.

An attempt should always be made to obtain at once efficient medical aid. The reduction of a dislocation, even within some hours, is not a matter of very great difficulty, but the trouble increases materially with lapse of time.

To give relief to suffering, and to prevent the occurrence of inflammation before the arrival of a medical man, the injured part may be treated by cold applications—local cold bathing, or the application of thin folds of linen wetted with cold water. Rest and support, as directed for a sprain, will also be available. Leeches in small numbers and applied frequently may be resorted to, and warm poultices or fomentations when they come off.

It is not possible to describe with unmistakeable clearness the several forms of dislocation, or the modes to be employed for their reduction; therefore, as a rule, the injury must be left alone, if medical aid cannot be had; but the patient may be very anxious that something should be done, and the dislocation may have happened more than once before. In this latter case, the injury will be much more easy to replace; and the patient, too, having a lively recollection of the means used on former occasions, will be able to speak of and to direct present manipulations.

These remarks apply with much force to *dislocations of the lower jaw.*

This is an unpleasing accident, and may occur on wide yawning, laughing, &c., to any one who has once had the accident before. The mouth is wide open and cannot be closed; the chin thrown forward; speech and swallowing very difficult; and in front of the ear there will be felt an unnatural hollow. *One* side only may be dislocated, and in this case the chin will be turned to the opposite side; *both* sides may be out of place and the chin will then be central.

The thumbs of the operator, protected with a napkin, should be placed within the mouth, in a line with, indeed, directly upon, the upper surfaces of the back teeth of the lower jaw; then he must press his thumbs downwards and backwards, while at the same moment he elevates the chin with the little and ring finger of each hand. If these movements are made with sufficient force and at the same moment, the jaw will slip into its place.

When reduction has been effected, the parts must be kept in comparative rest for some days. The patient should live on good soup, &c., or other food easily swallowed and not needing mastication, and the jaw should be supported by a cravat passed beneath it, so as to restrain movement, the ends of the cravat being tied at the top of the head.

Dislocation of the Shoulder Joint.

In this form of injury the arm-bone is displaced from its contact with the blade-bone. It is not uncommon; and having once occurred is very liable to happen again; under these conditions, too, the replacing the bone is not usually very difficult.

The arm in the most usual form of the accident cannot be moved without pain—the shoulder seems flattened, the elbow stands out from the side, cannot be made to touch the ribs, nor can it be brought up easily to a level with the shoulder; the head of the bone rounded in shape may be felt in the armpit, if the fingers are pushed well up while the arm is slightly moved outwards.

Reduction may be effècted in this mode. The operator sits on the edge of the bed on which the patient has been laid flat, and on the side corresponding to the injured joint. Having removed his boot, he should place the heel of the right foot in the patient's armpit, if the right shoulder be the one disabled, and *vice-versâ*, and then taking hold of the wrist with both hands he must pull steadily downwards, while the heel

98 FIRST HELP IN ACCIDENTS.

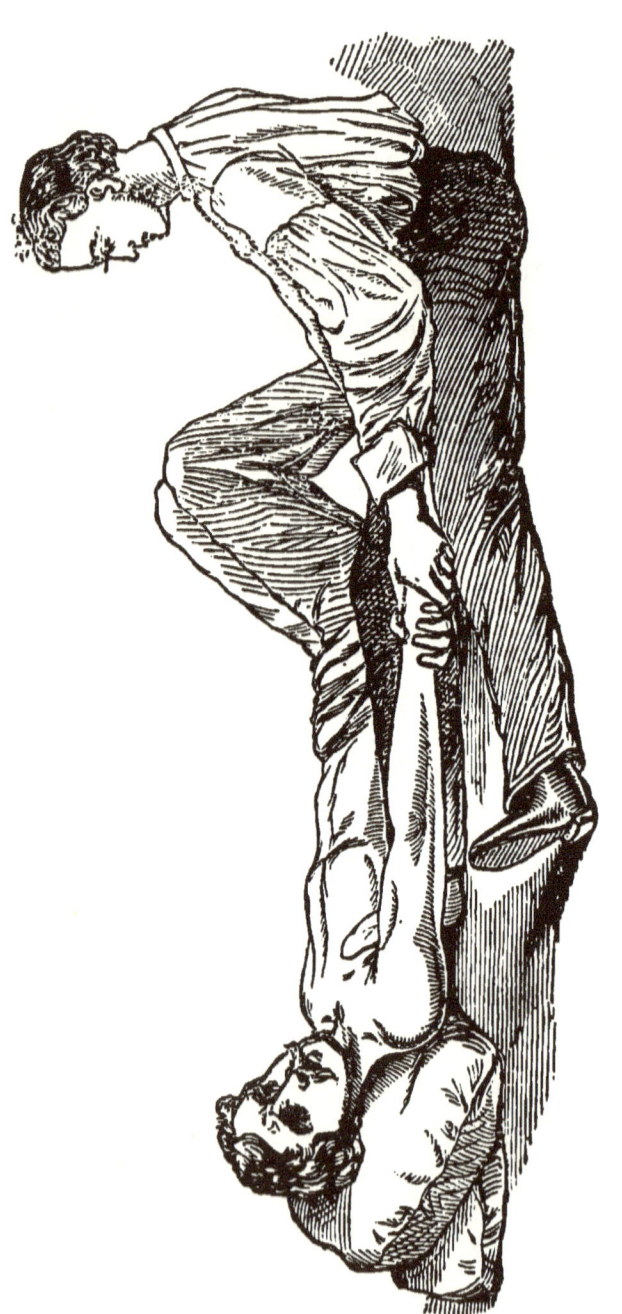

Fig. 20. Dislocation of Shoulder Joint.

fills up the armpit and forms a fixed point. The attention of the patient should be diverted by some question or exclamation, and after the extension has been continued for a little time, the head of the bone will most probably slip into its place without much difficulty.

Dislocation of the Thigh-bone at the Hip Joint.

The limb will be shortened and the toes turned in, so as to rest on the opposite foot, in the most ordinary form of this accident. If it has occurred more than once in the same person, it will be worth the trial to attempt the reduction on the same principles as those sketched out for the shoulder, the heel of the operator being well fixed in the fork, and extension made from the ankle or knee.

This plan can only succeed when the operator is taller and stronger than his patient. If the accident happen to a mus-

100   FIRST HELP IN ACCIDENTS.

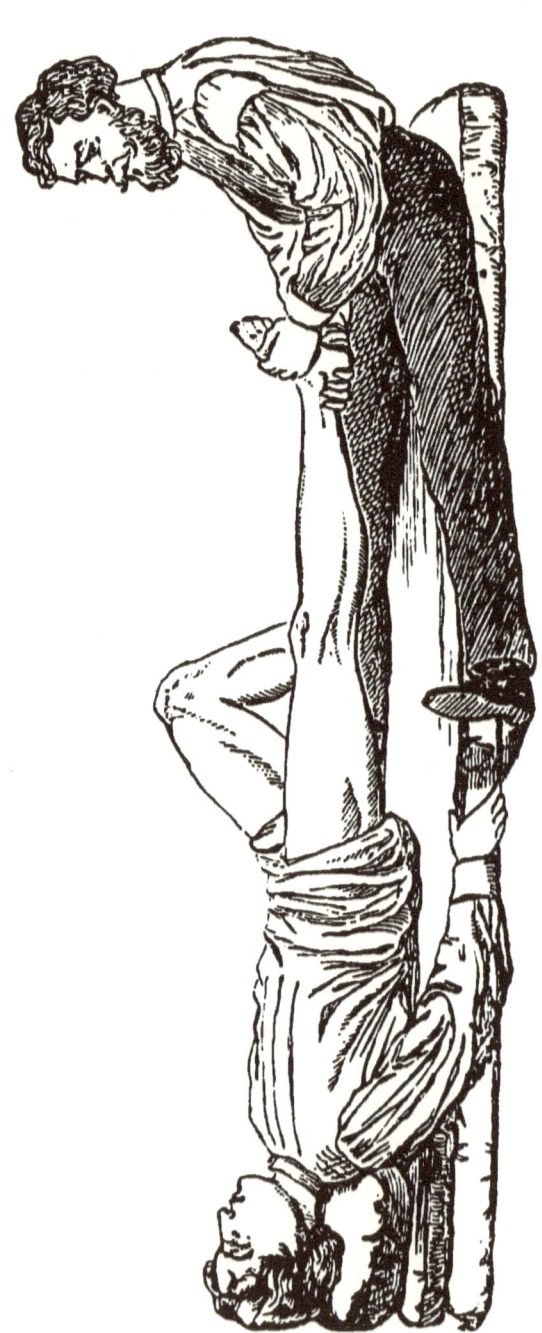

Fig. 21. Dislocation at Hip Joint.

cular man this mode of procedure may be tried :—

Pass a strong towel round the upper part of the thigh; fix this so that its direction of drawing is upwards and rather outwards; then extend the limb in a directly downward direction, by employing the muscular power of two or three assistants, who pull from a towel fixed round the limb, either just at the ankle or above the knee. The extension should be continued for some little time until the muscles of the limb are wearied, and then the head of the thigh-bone will probably slip in.

Displacement of the Internal Cartilage of the Knee Joint.

It may happen from an accidental twist of the leg in walking, or a fall with the leg bent underneath, that some injury is found to have happened to the knee. The patient cannot get his heel to the ground, is not unable to walk, but is obliged to walk on his toes, and with the knee slightly bent ;

the whole joint is not painful, and there is not at first much swelling — a tender point is found to exist on the inner face of the joint, and there may very well be a little puffiness here. The injury is really a *displacement of the plate of cartilage* which lies between the thigh-bone and the head of the leg-bone, and it may thus be rectified:—

Put the patient on his back on a mattress, bend the knee until the heel almost touches the buttock, and then, with one hand grasping the thigh firmly, and making pressure on the inner side of the knee, straighten the limb somewhat quickly and forcibly. The manœuvre may be repeated once or twice, but it will almost always succeed, and the patient can then walk as well as before the accident happened.

Subsequent rest for a short time, and the wearing of a bandage or knee-cap will be found advisable.

CHAPTER VIII.

FRACTURES, OR BROKEN BONES.

FRACTURES almost always result on violence directly or indirectly applied to the injured limb. The breaking happens generally at some distance from the joints, therefore in the length, or what is surgically termed the shaft of the bone.

It is not difficult to make out that fracture exists—there will be loss of power over the injured part more or less complete, some alteration in contour of the limb; it will be bent, twisted, or shortened; pain about the injured point, with swelling coming on even very quickly; and when the injured limb is moved by some bystander, there will be a freedom of motion which is not found in the healthy limb. Consequent on this very movement, too, especially if the fracture be about the middle of one of the long bones, there may very probably be heard a grating, due to the rubbing against one another of two irregular and roughened surfaces of bone.

All these signs may not be present; but if the limb have become suddenly powerless, and there be even some of the other symptoms, it will be wise to treat the case as if fracture had been declared to exist by a competent judge. It is difficult to give simple rules for the distinguishing between a fracture and a dislocation; in very many cases it is exceedingly difficult, but this much may be said:—

Fractures do not in the majority of cases implicate joints.

Dislocations have this as their especial character.

Again, the displacement of a fracture may generally, by a gentle and quiet extension, or drawing out of the limb, be remedied, and for the time, at least, the shortening and deformity will be found to disappear. Not so with a dislocation: this latter injury will require more forcible and more systematic extension.

The extreme mobility (in a bystander's hands) of the fractured ends, does not exist with the displacement of a bone at its articulation.

The position of the injured parts will vary too; a patient will have slightly moved his limb, if there is dislocation, to the most easy position; while the terminal part of a fractured limb will fall inwards or outwards merely by its own weight, and without reference to the patient's feelings of pain.

These injuries are usually met with when a person is dressed; therefore, unless there be bleeding, or something to call for immediate exposure and examination of the damaged part, do not be in a hurry to remove the clothes. If the arm be hurt, extemporize a sling from a neck-handkerchief or some other article of dress, and support the arm from elbow to wrist, tying the ends of the handkerchief in a knot over the coat-collar behind. If the thigh or leg be in pain, fasten the injured limb to its fellow by a cravat-bandage or two, and take care that they lie side by side, and on the same level; or fasten outside the clothes some temporary support, a piece or two of straight stick with a bandage, and then remove the sufferer quietly and carefully to some house near at hand.

If medical aid be available, send for it without any delay; and be careful, if in the country, and so at some distance from the doctor's house, to forward a clear statement as to the apparent nature of the accident, which limb is hurt, and where, and how it happened; let this statement, too, be in writing, if possible.

It may well happen, however, that skilled assistance cannot be had, and in this case the patient should be undressed quietly and cautiously. It will be far better to slit up the dress on the arm or leg with a pair of scissors than to pull it off; but however the uncovering of the injury may be managed, it must be done very slowly and gently, and the limb should be supported so as to prevent jarring or shaking to the damaged part; it must be carefully kept, too, in a right direction, for otherwise some sharp splinter of bone may penetrate the hitherto unwounded skin.

Fractures have received various names in accordance with the characters they present; for our present purpose, it will be sufficient to speak of them as—

Simple or Compound.—A *simple* fracture is the term applied to the injury, where the bone is broken, but with no co-existing external wound of the integument; while the name of *compound* refers to those fractures where there is external laceration of the skin, and a wound leading down, in the majority of instances, directly to the broken ends of the bone. In the main points of treatment there is but little difference; the *simple* fracture will heal much the more quickly of the two; and the *compound* injury will be most successfully treated by those means which will tend to the immediate healing of the wound of the skin, and so to the exclusion of the outer air from the interior injury. If there be much laceration of the skin, from the bone having protruded through it, or from the force or direction of the first injury, the wound must be treated as a severe lacerated wound, with water-dressing, poultices, &c.; but if the external aperture be a small one, and the edges of this small wound not battered or bruised, it may be closed at once by putting over it a piece of lint dipped in blood or soaked with Friar's balsam, then leaving this dressing undisturbed as long as possible.

In order to treat fractures successfully, the attention should be directed to the following points:—

1. To insure the fitting together of the fractured parts.

2. To maintain the ends in close apposition.

3. To keep the sufferer in a state of thorough quietude, if the fracture involve the principal bone or bones of a limb.

New reparative material is thrown out very speedily, between and around the ends of the breakage, and subsequently becomes converted into bone. A period varying from one to three months will be required for the thorough repair of the damage, according to the locality and severity of the wound; the time will vary, too, according to the supply of blood usually afforded to the part. Thus, fractures about the face or trunk are repaired more speedily than those of the limbs.

As already named in an earlier chapter, splints, or unyielding pieces of material, and bandages are essential to the successful treatment. Pads of soft stuff may be with advantage introduced between the splints and the limb, with the purpose of transmitting an equally diffused and constant support, and of preventing undue pressure on any prominent point.

Pain and swelling are the immediate or early results of a fracture, and it is well that a non-professional, in undertaking a case, should allow several hours, it may be even a day or two, to pass over before he ventures to apply the splints and rollers as a permanent dressing. Yet the limb must not be left quite alone. Lateral support should be given to it by small pillows, pads of tow, folded garments, or some such soft materials, and cold applications, lint dipped in cold water, &c., will aid in removing the swelling. If the leg or thigh be broken, the limb may be placed in its proper direction on one or more long pillows, and these tied at intervals round the limb with some tapes or cravat bandages.

The subsequent treatment, the swelling

and pain having in some measure at least subsided, may thus be managed:—

1. Well wash the limb with some soap and water and a large sponge; some weeks must pass before this can again be done; dry with a soft towel, then,

2. Gently, yet firmly, draw the limb down into its normal position, so doing away with the alteration in shape. Gentle pressure about the seat of injury will aid in putting the fragments (there may be several such pieces) in their proper position. Let the limb be held in this form by some second person until—

3. Splints can be applied. They are best made of wood, cut a little wider and longer than the division of the limb where the injury has been inflicted, and should have some soft pads on their inside: these last may be formed from tow or cotton wool, stitched up in folds of linen—from pieces of flannel, soft carpeting, or woollen structures cut to the size of the splints,

and placed in the requisite number of folds and thickness. The splints must be retained in close contact with the limb, by cravat bandages, straps fitted with buckles, or by rollers applied as directed in a previous section.

Pasteboard or gutta-percha will afford ready means for the making splints for fractures, especially of the smaller bones, simply needing to be softened in hot water; they will assume very fairly the shape of any part to which they are applied, and therefore should be fitted when the fracture has been reduced, and while the parts are still retained by the operator's hands in the required position.

A satisfactory casing, combining the firmness of more solid material with the ease of application of an ordinary roller, may be had from the use of rollers soaked in starch of usual consistence, or in a mixture of acacia-gum mucilage, thickened with chalk. The limb should first be covered throughout with wadding retained in place by a dry roller, and upon this the starch roller well soaked may be applied, taking care to make the turns evenly, and to place each turn closely on the preceding one. In a few hours it will be dry and firm.

This mode of dressing is available for a non-professional in simple fractures of one or even of the two bones either of fore arm or leg; and as a subsequent protection, when the splints, &c., first applied have been removed, therefore at the expiration of three or four weeks.

Certain fractures demand a special notice :—

1. *Fractures of the Ribs* are consequent on a fall or severe blow on the side. There is complaint of aching pain, which becomes acute on deep inspiration, and is referred to one particular point, and very commonly, on applying the fingers to this point, grating may be felt as the patient breathes.

They are best treated by the use of a flannel bandage four or five fingers' breadth so applied in turns round the chest as to give support to the injured part, and to limit the movements of the chest-walls in breathing. *Or,* the affected side may be strapped up with broad and long strips of soap plaster, one overlapping the preceding one, but leaving the uninjured side quite free from restraint. Where this latter plan can be managed it will be preferable. Each strip of plaster should reach from the centre of the chest to the middle line of the spinal column behind.

Subsequent acute pain may require smart lowering measures — low diet and bleeding.

2. *Fracture of the Collar-bone.* — This injury mostly results upon a fall when the person has struck the shoulder violently on the ground, *e.g.,* in fall from horseback; but it may be caused by direct violence to the bone itself.

There is a feeling of loss of support to the corresponding arm; it cannot be raised to the level of the shoulder without a good deal of pain; there will be projection of one end or the other at the seat of fracture, the one piece of bone thus overlapping the other one, and grating may be felt on pressure with the fingers. If both shoulders be drawn backwards at the same moment, this overlapping of the fractured ends will disappear.

The simplest mode of treating this injury is by the use of three handkerchiefs —large square ones will be best for the purpose. Of these, one should be folded tightly into the shape of a square pad and placed well up into the armpit, so as to keep the shoulder up and out; another put on as a sling, embracing in its hold the whole fore-arm from the elbow to the wrist; and the third employed for the purpose of retaining the arm in close contact with the side of the chest.

If a long and broad roller be within reach, it may be used to confine the arm to the chest in place of the third handkerchief. The handkerchiefs and roller should

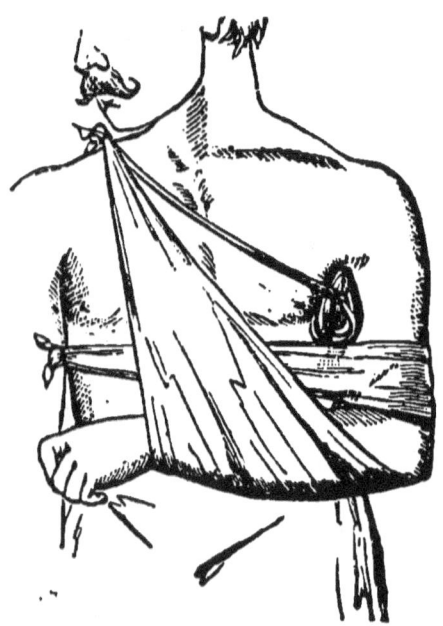

Fig. 22. Fracture of Collar-bone.

be firmly stitched together, more especially at the points where they intersect, with the purpose of preventing slipping.

The arm should be retained in its immovable position for three weeks or a month, and some thickening or elevation must be expected to remain at the site of fracture, from the difficulty of maintaining the fragments perfectly in place.

The figure of 8 bandage may be employed in the treatment of this fracture, so that each terminal loop embraces and draws backwards the shoulders, while the layers of bandage will cross each other at the middle of the back, just between the bladebones. Possibly this will secure more perfect fitting of the fragments, but it is certainly more irksome to the patient. A sling will in this case also be advisable.

3. *Fracture of the Upper Arm.* — The patient is unable to bend the elbow or raise the fore-arm, and there will be the usual signs of fracture at the point where pain is felt. As a rule, the injury results in some direct violence.

The arm-bone (humerus) may be fractured at any point between its ends. The following remarks will only apply to a simple fracture occurring about the middle of the shaft.

A roller should be put on from the fingers upwards, covering the whole limb to the shoulder, and the arm is best placed with the elbow bent at a right angle. Then four splints should be provided, two rather longer than the third and fourth. These will be best made of wood, and of a width proportioned

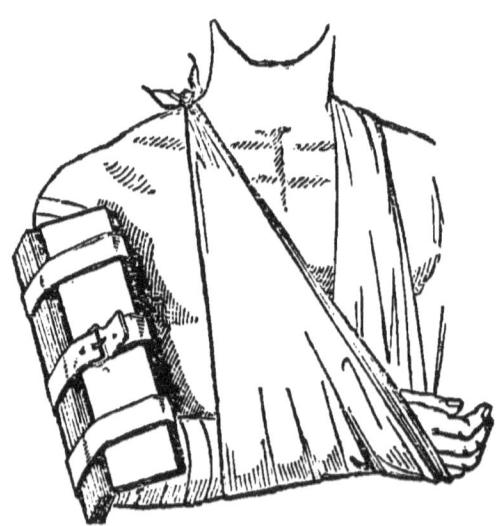

Fig. 23. Fracture of Upper Arm

to the size of the arm. Each splint should have a soft pad of tow wrapped in linen, or some folds of flannel on its inside. Then one splint, the longest, should be placed outside from the shoulder to the elbow; another almost equally long on the back surface of the arm to the point of the elbow; while the third and fourth are placed on the inside and front of the arm. Care must be taken that the fourth and shortest splint, reaching from the bend of the elbow to the armpit, does not press too much on these points: the ends of the pad should cover over the extremities of the splint. These splints, so applied as to embrace and steady the fracture, should be retained in position by two or three webbing straps with buckles, or by a roller evenly and carefully applied. A sling will serve to support the fore-arm, and the patient should, if possible, sit up in preference to lying down: in the former position the mere weight of the fore-arm tends to keep the fractured ends better in their place.

4. *Fracture of the Fore-Arm.*—The alteration of shape and the inability to perform movements without pain, will with other symptoms of fracture tell the existence of this injury. Of the two bones one only may be broken; this will not be easily detected, but the uninjured bone will almost obviate the need for casing the fracture with splints. Supposing that both

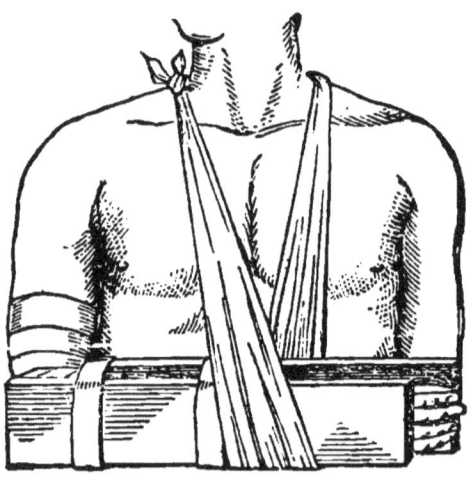

Fig. 24. Fracture of Fore-Arm.

bones are fractured, two padded splints will be necessary, reaching from the tips of the fingers to the point of the elbow, one placed before, the other behind — only taking care that the fore-arm is so placed, after the fracture has been adjusted and before the splints are fixed, that the inside of the hand and fore-arm looks directly to the front of the chest. The splints will need securing with roller or webbing straps, and a sling wider than in fig. 24, more spread out from wrist to elbow, will also be necessary.

5. *Fracture of the Thigh* follows generally on direct violence, and may occur at any point throughout the shaft of the bone. It is not difficult to detect; usually there is some shortening, positive alteration in contour, and the patient is unable to raise his limb from the bed.

It may be treated by using the sound limb as a splint, thus :—The patient should be placed flat on his back, and the injured limb be quietly and firmly drawn down by traction at the ankle until it corresponds in length with the opposite limb. Then the two limbs must be fastened together at knee and ankle by webbing-band, or with buckle, or by turns of a broad roller; first, however, taking care that at all possible points of contact some well-made pads intervene between the two limbs, therefore especially at the sides of the feet, the ankles, and the knees. The patient must be kept quiet in bed for six weeks at least.

The application, however, of a long splint on the outside of the limb, with a shorter splint on the inside, will furnish the best security for satisfactory repair of the broken bone. For an adult the splints should be about four fingers' breadth, and well padded with flannel, or layers of tow encased in linen or calico. The outer one will vary in length according to the height of the patient; it should project some four inches below the foot, and reach up to midway between the outer and upper prominence of the thigh-bone (great trochanter) and the armpit.

FRACTURES.

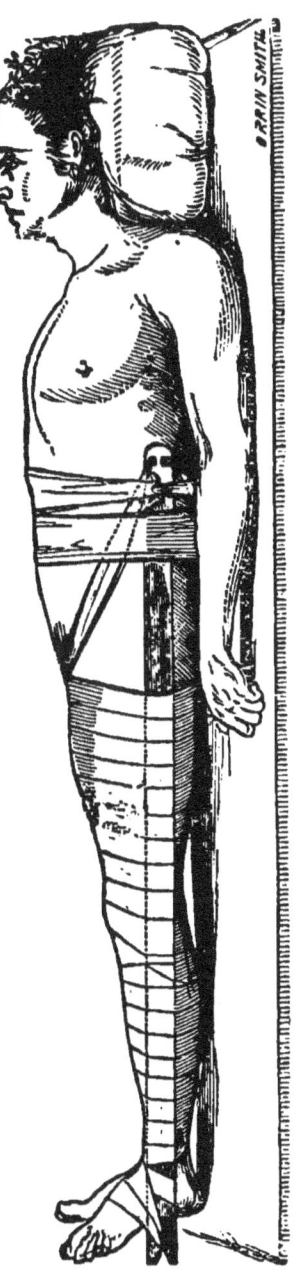

Fig. 25. Fracture of Thigh

First, then, the whole limb should be evenly bandaged from toes to groin; then the outer splint will need applying, and the limb must be firmly fastened to it.

It is customary to have two deep notches cut at the lower extremity of the piece of board, and two holes bored through it close to the upper end. The foot must be fixed to the lower end of the splint, carrying the roller round the ankle and instep, and then after each turn through the notches just mentioned — extra padding, cotton, wool, or tow, will be needed to protect the prominences of the outer and inner ankle from too much pressure. Then the limb to a little above the knee must be bandaged to the splint; and this point reached, the upper end of the splint must be fixed so as to prevent shortening at the fractured point, by passing a folded handkerchief round the groin, the two ends of which may be threaded through the holes at the upper extremity of the splint and firmly knotted. Instead of the pocket-handkerchief a roller may be used. The inner splint, reaching only from inside of knee to the groin, may now be put on, and the roller carried upwards so as to encircle the whole, and retain both splints in close contact with the injured thigh.

Rollers or pocket-handkerchiefs should fasten the splint to the abdomen, the knot of the latter being made upon the splint.

The patient must of necessity lie on his back, and six or eight weeks will pass over before the fracture is thoroughly consolidated.

6. *Fracture of the Leg.*—The two bones of the leg may be broken at the same time, or one only may be fractured. If the latter be the case, it is usually the outside and more slender one of the two that is broken across, and for this little treatment is necessary.

If both bones are broken the patient is

unable to raise his limb; there is distortion and swelling, with pain at the seat of fracture, and the ends of the bones will move on one another slightly if the limb be raised by an assistant.

The fracture may be treated by the employment of two side splints: these should be applied well padded, one to each side of the limb, and retained in place by webbing straps or by roller. The patient should then lie on his side, the one corresponding with the fracture, keeping the limb as immovable as possible. Four

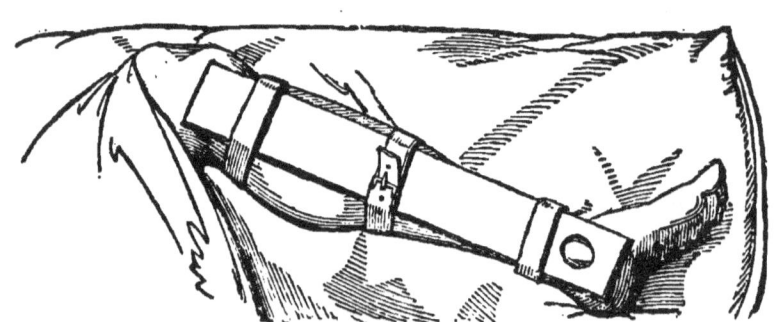

Fig. 26. Fracture of the Leg.

or five weeks' confinement to bed must be insisted on.

Or, again, the patient may have the less irksome position on his back, if the fractured limb be steadied either by *a straight outside splint,* or by the application of *moulded splints combined with starch or gum and chalk casing.*

If the straight outside splint be employed, it should be made of wood four fingers' breadth, to reach from the knee to below the foot, and with the lower end notched as in the long thigh splint. The inequalities about the ankle are great, so that the padding must be abundant and well arranged; the limb must be well fixed to the splint by roller, put on as directed in the case of a thigh fracture.

Should the moulded splints be preferred, the limb is first to be covered with a dry roller; upon this closely fitted to the limb, while they are still pliable from soaking in hot water, gutta-percha or pasteboard splints may be adapted; and these will form a satisfactory basis for the application over them of a bandage thoroughly soaked in starch of the consistence of cream, or in a mixture of the mucilage of acacia-gum into which chalk has been stirred to afford some consistence. This wetted bandage should be put on just as any ordinary roller, very evenly and closely, and the composition, starch, &c., should be well smeared over the whole outside of the roller, so as to cover over and cement down each successive turn. If the limb so encased be exposed to the air, it will in a few hours have a thoroughly firm and continuous support from one end to the other. This plan of treatment will allow the patient more and earlier freedom of movement than he could dare to use with the older form of splints.

In the remarks above given with respect to fractures of the lower extremity, it may be well to mention that in each instance a careful adjustment of the fracture is presupposed before any apparatus can be applied. Firm yet steady drawing down of the limb by the operator, while an assistant fixes the bony framework about the hips, will procure the necessary length; and gentle pressure on the displaced fragments will mould the immediate neighbourhood of the damaged bone to something like its natural form. This having been done, the limb must be retained in its improved position by the hands of some competent bystander until splints and bandages can be applied.

All these measures must be carried out without absolute force. Quiet and gentle proceedings will accomplish far more than any exertion of main strength.

7. *Fractures of the bones about the head and face* may occur: it is not possible that a non-professional can treat them satisfactorily with the intention of replacing fragments, &c. All that is open to him is to insist on thorough rest of the parts, to apply cold and soothing applications, and

to remove any foreign material that may be lodged in the wounds inflicted at the same time. An exception to these remarks may exist in—

8. *Fracture of the Lower Jaw.* — This injury is not difficult of detection: it results on direct violence, and the bone in its whole outline is so easily examined by the fingers that irregularity or change of direction must be found out. Sometimes it will be enough to support the injured bone, if there be but little displacement, by one or more cravat bandages, which are applied so as to retain the jaw in place, and may be tied one at the back of the neck, and another across the top of the head. If, however, there be separation and displacement, such that the two ends cannot easily be maintained on the same plane, a further arrangement must be contrived; and this will be best done by employing a piece of gutta-percha, moulded so as to form a cover for the jaw on both sides, and

in its whole length; this will give some defined support, and may be kept in place by the use of cravat bandages, or a roller applied as above directed. Some three weeks will pass before union can be looked for; and through this period the patient should be constantly supported on soups, beef-tea, &c., &c.

It is imperative that when a fracture of the lower extremity has been reduced and secured by splints, the limb should be protected from accidental catching of the bed clothes, &c., which might cause sudden jerks of the limb and lead to severe pain. The clothes should be kept away by using some stools, or, better still, cradles: these are made either of wicker or wood in the shape of an arch, and represent exactly one-half of a circle, the free edges resting on the bed. The limb should be placed in the vacant space between the two sides, and so under the arch.

One word may be added respecting the mode of dealing with fractures which extend into or are in close proximity to joints. It will happen, not unfrequently

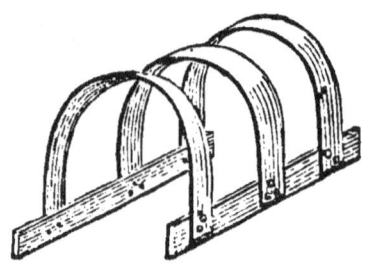

Fig. 27. Cradle.

under the most favourable conditions of attendance and care, that the joint implicated in the injury remains ever afterwards stiff and fixed. This result must be expected, and therefore the fractured ends should be placed in close apposition to ensure union as directed in the above sections, while the joint is straightened or bent at such an angle as may be most convenient for after use, remembering that in this position once chosen, the limb will probably remain for the rest of life.

Therefore, if the fracture have happened in the lower extremity, and the knee-joint be involved in the injury, the knee must be nearly straightened, so that walking may be afterwards accomplished with but little trouble. If fracture extend into the ankle-joint, the foot must be placed at right angles to the leg.

The elbow may be implicated, and then in accordance with the employment or the wishes of the patient, the fore-arm should be placed at an angle more or less decided with the upper arm ; probably as a rule the angle should be rather more than a right angle.

CHAPTER IX.

OF THE LODGMENT OF FOREIGN BODIES IN THE THROAT, IN THE GULLET, OR IN THE AIR PASSAGES.

THE foreign bodies with which one may have to deal as causing obstructions in the throat and gullet are usually derived from food taken into the mouth. A piece of half-masticated meat may stick in the throat between the arches of the palate, or may be arrested from its bulk as it passes down the gullet. The involuntary efforts to swallow which are excited by the presence of this mass only serve to increase the evil, and unless relief be afforded actual suffocation may result from this simple accident.

The first rule should be to place the

patient where a good light can fall from a window or a lamp into his mouth, and then boldly and quickly examine the back of the throat and the base of the tongue by passing the fore-finger well down—very possibly the foreign mass may be touched at once and extracted by the fingers with comparative ease. The procedure will be facilitated by first directing that the tongue be put forward well out of the mouth, and there retained, being grasped by the patient's own fingers covered with a handkerchief. This manœuvre mechanically draws forward the arches of the palate, and allows the operator to sweep his finger well across from one side to the other of the throat.

A fish-bone may be the offending body, and this may be caught and extracted in the same mode. No pincers or forceps are half so good for the purpose as the finger and thumb of a resolute bystander, who knows what he has to do and has nerve to do it.

But the mass may have gone lower down,

quite into the canal of the œsophagus, and there, although it will not produce such marked symptoms, or threaten danger to life by arrest of breathing, it will still produce great discomfort. If a piece of meat of some size be so lodged, the drinking copious draughts of water and swallowing them rapidly will very possibly cause it to pass on into the stomach. Should this fail, it may be well to try the effect of an inverted action, and attempt to expel the mass by producing vomiting. For this purpose the patient must take an emetic; and the safest compound is the sulphate of zinc, dissolving twenty grains of this in a small quantity of warm water for a single dose. This quantity of the salt may be repeated in ten minutes, and vomiting will almost certainly follow speedily. In the absence of this drug, common salt, or mustard dissolved in water, or olive oil may be resorted to to serve the same end.

If vomiting fails to eject the plug from

the gullet, it is imperative that mechanical means be tried for its removal, but these should be intrusted only to a medical man. If, however, it be impossible to obtain skilled assistance the operator may obtain a slip of whalebone, and tie firmly to one end of it a knob of sponge about the size of a marble. This will form an extempore probang, and it may be thus used:—The patient should throw his head well back, and put the tongue out while the operator introduces the probang, sponge end first, into the throat, so as to touch the further wall, and then pushes it on down the gullet so as to displace and send before it the foreign mass into the stomach.

Fish-bones or pins caught in the gullet may be treated by swallowing some pulpy mass—masticated bread, &c.—so that this may entangle and carry onwards the sharp-pointed substance.

Under none of the above conditions should medical assistance be neglected—

the cases even in the slighter forms need prompt and skilled attention. More serious instances occur where irregular and awkwardly shaped substances—a plate with artificial teeth, for example—can only be extracted by a surgical operation.

Foreign bodies may take a different course and make their way into some portion of the air passages, there exciting much more disturbance than if they had passed into the gullet. If they lie simply across the throat at the entrance of the larynx, it will be sometimes possible to remove them by the finger and thumb introduced as above directed; more frequently, however, it is found that the substances pass on into the larynx, the organ for the production of voice sounds, or into the windpipe and its divisions. The symptoms of such an accident will be unmistakeable; local pain, soreness, difficulty of breathing, with continual harsh cough, ending not impossibly in the production of acute inflammation and subsequent death. It will rarely be possible to procure the expulsion of any foreign body when it has once fairly entered the air passages, except by the surgical operation of opening the larynx or windpipe; when the artificial wound is made sufficiently large the substance will usually be coughed up, or it may be removed by forceps.

This remedial measure can only be carried out by a surgeon; and if such skilled aid cannot be obtained, the removal of the offending material can hardly be looked for. In some few instances the following means have proved effectual :—

Fasten the patient firmly to the seat and back of a common strong chair, so that by fastening cords to the chair and running them over a pulley or beam, it will be possible to invert the individual head downwards, at all events for a few seconds at a time. The chest or back may at the same time be smartly knocked, so as mechanically to dislodge if possible the impacted substance. Much will of course depend upon the size of the foreign body and the position which it may have reached; but the plan has been so far successful, that it is, to say the least of it, quite worthy of a careful and prolonged trial. It is not possible that a non-professional person could successfully carry out the operation of opening the windpipe.

CHAPTER X.

OF POISONING.

POISONOUS compounds may be introduced into the body by various routes, not only by the natural openings, but also by applications to the skin, by inhalation of vapours, &c. According to the different character of the poisons, so will the symptoms resulting on their reception into the system essentially differ. These will be briefly noted further on: it may be well now to mention some of the main rules which will lead to the suspicion of poisoning; these may afford assistance in the immediate treatment to any intelligent reader, but medical aid in any case of poisoning should be obtained, if possible. No rules can be laid down for the satisfactory after treatment: this is only effectually to be carried out by professional knowledge.

If poison has been taken, the symptoms appear suddenly while the person is in health.

The symptoms appear, too, soon after a meal, or within some short time after the taking either of food or medicine. This condition is only valuable where the introduction of the poisonous agent by the skin, by inhalation, &c., is by other circumstances excluded.

If several persons partake of the same meal, and the food contain poison, all must be expected to suffer in the same way.

The noxious agent may be discovered in the food taken, or in the matters vomited.

The above four statements are, with certain limitations, such as coincident illness, &c., to be taken into consideration in inquiring into and treating a case of suspected poisoning: thus poisons do not lie dormant in the system for several hours before their effect is produced, nor are there many diseases which affect the system by sudden invasion, without some premonitory indications of disturbed health.

Using the term poisoning in its wide sense, the following classes, into which for convenience injurious materials may be divided, will embrace the most usual manifestations :—

I.—*Irritant Poisons :—*
Such are—
1. *Acids.*—Sulphuric acid (oil of vitriol), nitric acid (aquafortis), hydrochloric acid (spirit of salt); these, too, of vegetable origin, oxalic, acetic, and tartaric acids.
2. *Alkalies.*—Potash, soda, ammonia, and their carbonates.
3. *Metallic Compounds.*—Arsenic, arsenious acid, mercury, lead, copper, zinc, &c., &c., together with some of their more soluble salts.

4. *Vegetable Irritants.*—Aloes, gamboge, &c., &c.

II.—*Narcotic Poisons :*—

1. Opium, prussic acid, henbane, &c.
2. Alcohol in any of its common forms; wine, spirits, malt liquors, &c.
3. As vapours inhaled and so affecting the system. Carbonic acid, sulphuretted hydrogen, chloroform, &c.

III.—*Animal Poisons. Poisoned Wounds,* &c. Wounds from bites of mad dogs, snake bites, &c.

IV.—*Animal Poisons as taken into the system* by tainted or decomposed meat, bad fish, sausages, &c.

V.—*Accidental swallowing of noxious things*—such as leeches, Spanish flies, &c., &c.

The above list might be subdivided and so rendered more true and more complete;

but the simple form will give sufficiently clear data for action in a case of emergency from the taking of poison, and in the absence of medical advice.

TREATMENT OF POISONING.

§ 1. *General Remarks.*

If there be the certainty that poison has been taken, the measures for relief must be put in practice without any delay. Even a few minutes more or less may make the turning-point of saving or losing life, and therefore even though medical assistance have been sent for at once, the attendant will be thoroughly justified in commencing that plan of treatment which may appear to him the most judicious.

To some of the poisons direct chemical antidotes can be found, the resulting compound being, if not indeed absolutely without influence on the human stomach, far less noxious than the original dose. Fortunately, these counter poisons can be found in almost every household, and they should be given at once.

Others, again, of the substances in the list just given are best prevented from causing serious injury, by the prompt procuring of free vomiting. This may be effected by mechanically tickling the back of the throat with a feather, by large draughts of warm salt and water, or warm mustard and water; and more satisfactorily still by an emetic of ipecacuanha wine, one or two tablespoonsful for a dose, or by the dissolving in a wineglass of warm water some twenty or thirty grains of sulphate of zinc, repeating any of these emetic draughts once or more until the full effect is produced. Do not give the antimonial preparations, tartar emetic, &c.; they are far too depressing in their action, and not well under control.

It may be, however, that neither by chemical action nor by vomiting can the poison well be dealt with, and in these conditions the attempt may be made to diminish the local action upon the walls of the stomach, &c., by the use of mucilaginous and oily drinks, which may envelop the noxious material, and in a measure lessen the resulting damage — such, for instance, as milk, barley-water, white of eggs, salad oil, &c. Any of these draughts are well available for this purpose.

These soothing and demulcent things are also well suited for the treatment of the after stages of the irritation, when the poison has been in great measure removed or neutralized.

The patient, after he may have escaped the first imminent danger, will undergo great risk from the subsequent changes which follow in the stomach, &c., on the taking of the poison. It is only possible for a non-professional to treat such a state by soothing remedies, slops, &c.; to insist on thorough quietude, and to relieve internal pain by the external and frequent application of hot poultices, fomentations, or mustard plasters. The food should be very plain and simple, and given rather very frequently than in large quantities.

§ 2. SPECIAL RULES FOR TREATMENT OF THE DIFFERENT KINDS OF POISONS.

I.—*Irritant Poisons.*

1. If *acids* have been taken, it is not difficult to find a direct antidote near at hand.

The local action on the lips, mouth, and throat, will usually leave little doubt as to the agent which has been swallowed. Sulphuric acid chars and blackens the tissues; nitric and hydrochloric acids equally destroy the parts they are in contact with, leaving respectively a yellowish or whitish condition of the damaged textures.

No emetic treatment is in this case to be

attempted; indeed, the poison itself, from its intense local action, will bring on severe retching and attempts at vomiting. The *alkalies* are the appropriate remedies: soda or potash dissolved in water and given freely. In their absence, the ordinary carbonate of magnesia, or Dinneford's solution, may be used, or common whiting or chalk suspended in water will answer the same good purpose. These should be administered in repeated draughts for some little time, and followed by some mucilaginous and soothing fluid—such as milk or barley-water.

2. For the treatment of poisoning by the *alkalies, potash, soda,* &c., *acids* must be employed. The most readily obtained will be ordinary vinegar, best diluted with half its bulk of water; citric or tartaric acid, also dissolved in water. Lemon-juice or beer if at all acid may be employed.

Soothing and demulcent remedies should be employed, after the poison has been fairly neutralized by the acid mixtures.

3. The antidotes for *metallic poisons* must be chosen according to the special substance which has been swallowed. As a rule, however, the attempt to provoke vomiting may well be made by the administration of an emetic of sulphate of zinc.

If *arsenic* has been taken, a mixture of milk and lime-water or soda-water in equal parts should be freely drunk. Light magnesia diffused in water may be taken. Vomiting and retching will most probably follow on the taking of the poison; if not, as there will be much irritation of the stomach, emetics are best avoided. There is some reason to believe that common animal charcoal has sometimes at least been of service, and this might be tried.

Corrosive Sublimate.—The bichloride of mercury is most speedily and best treated by the giving the albumen or white part of eggs and copious draughts of milk. In the absence of eggs, flour mixed with water may be given.

Acetate or Sugar of Lead. — The best remedy here is to give sulphuric acid (oil of vitriol), largely diluted with water, or as an emetic and antidote in one the sulphate of zinc in the dose before named.

It would be impossible to enumerate in small space the various metallic poisons; most of them, however, call for immediate emetics and treatment in some one of the above-mentioned modes.

4. *Vegetable irritants* may be treated by an early emetic, and by demulcent drinks: as a rule, they expend themselves by over excessive action on the intestinal canal.

II.—*Narcotic or Stupefying Poisons.*

Such as—

1. *Opium and its various preparations.* —The treatment should commence by the removal from the stomach, by a smart emetic, of any part of the poison yet

remaining there. The symptoms will be those of intense drowsiness, going on to heavy sleep, insensibility, and death, if much of the poisonous compound have entered into the circulation.

After an emetic, the pouring of cold water from some little height upon the head, neck, and shoulders is often of service in rousing the patient; then apply mustard poultices to the calves of the legs or to the feet. If the patient can swallow, give him hot and strong coffee, and expose him without hesitation to a free current of air. He may be able to walk, and if so, supported on each side, he should be kept moving, walking to and fro until the drowsiness has passed off, and he can sit down without going to sleep.

To children, more especially, even very small doses of opium are dangerous; the same treatment as named above should be used, combined with continuous friction of the limbs with warm flannels; placing the child in a hot bath, and then sponging with cold water—anything, in short, that will serve the purpose of keeping up respiration to its normal condition, and of preventing sleep and stupor.

2. *Prussic Acid.*—If in *small* doses, ammonia or strong coffee may be given; cold affusion upon the head and chest afterwards, rubbing dry with warm towels and free access of air. These means are most likely to be of use, and may be vigorously put in practice to save life.

If in *large* doses, no kind of treatment will be of any good; death happens in a very short time, even though medical aid may chance to be close at hand.

The treatment named above for opium poisoning will be advisable for similar symptoms, consequent on the taking of other vegetable sedatives.

3. *Alcohol* taken into the stomach acts first as an excitant, and subsequently as a decided narcotic poison. It is possible

to produce these effects by any of the compounds usually drunk; they follow, however, more rapidly when the poison is received into the system in some concentrated form. Spirits act more rapidly than wines or ale, &c.

Insensibility may come on after a large dose of undiluted spirit very speedily indeed. More frequently the stage of coma or stupor is only reached by degrees.

This condition is treated by the evacuation of the stomach, and by the employment of such remedies as will rouse the nervous system. Hot and strong coffee, externally applied stimuli, and frictions perseveringly carried on, are the most reliable means. The warmth of the body must be steadily kept up.

4. *Narcotism* may be caused by the inhaling of certain gases, &c.: the lungs are as effectual channels for the passage of poisons into the system as the stomach and intestinal canal. Alcohol can induce

drunkenness by long exposure to its fumes alone; and chloroform is a striking instance of a thoroughly sedative vapour.

The condition is a thorough poisoning; yet, in compliance with the popular impression, the poisonings by inhaling of gases, &c., will be noticed in Chapter XI., under the head of Suffocation.

III.—*Animal Poisons.—Poisoned Wounds.*

Animal poisons may be introduced into the system by the *stings of insects*. The sting of a wasp or bee may be visible, and if so, it should be extracted without delay; then apply to the wound a strong solution of ammonia in spirit or in water. In the absence of this agent, warm oil may be used. The same application of warm oil is much to be relied on in the stings or bites of tropical insects. There is commonly, too, general depression of the heart's action, with faintness, after severe stings; and to meet this some stimulant, brandy and water, for example, may be freely given.

Snake-bites are most successfully treated by the free use of stimulants, to counteract the excessive prostration, with the local use of warm oil well rubbed into and around the injured point. It would seem that cauterizing the point where the fang has entered with nitric acid, or with an iron heated to a white heat, has been of service in some cases in preventing the advance of alarming symptoms.

The Bite of a Mad Dog is the exciting cause of that fearful disease, hydrophobia. It is quite impossible that the treatment of the affection once fairly developed, can be canvassed in these pages. All that the subject admits of here is to insist strongly on the necessity of *preventive* measures.

If a person has been bitten by a dog, and there be any reason to believe the dog mad, have the part *at once* attended to. It may, if in a very exposed part, be possible to cut out with one sweep of a penknife the whole track of the animal's tooth; should a finger be bitten and torn much, it would be wise to chop the finger off at once, or cut it off at the knuckle with a knife. If the bite be in a part where cutting is not so easy, the only plan left is to burn the whole line of the wound thoroughly by introducing a knitting needle, heated previously to a white heat, to the very bottom of the opening, so destroying the tissues with which the animal's saliva has been brought into direct contact. As a means almost as effectual, but not so thoroughly active, the stick of nitrate of silver may be pushed to every point of the wound, yet of the two the actual cautery is far to be preferred.

Decomposing animal matter from hides, &c., has been found to cause a chain of very serious symptoms, and even death. To insure these consequences, it seems imperative that the poison must be applied to some, however slightly abraded surface, so that absorption into the system may take place. Severe erysipelatous inflammation about and around the part affected soon sets in, with formation of large collections of matter, and the patient very probably sinks, from the depression and damage to his constitutional powers.

If such a case should occur away from the possibility of obtaining medical aid, the nonprofessional must administer an abundance of wine and nourishment, and if matter come near the surface, it should be let out by a free incision.

IV.—*Animal Poisons taken into the System. —Bad Food.*

Animal Poisons may again be received into the system through eating decomposed or tainted meat, sausages, &c.

The symptoms are usually those of an

irritant poison : pain about the stomach, severe purging, and sometimes vomiting.

The offending material should be ejected from the stomach by the action of a sharp emetic, and the remaining symptoms must be treated by the application of external warmth, hot flannels on which some turpentine has been sprinkled, mustard poultices, &c. The appropriate remedies must be used, if there should be well-marked faintness or depression.

V.—*Accidental swallowing of noxious things.*

It may happen that *leeches* are swallowed in drinking water from some impure source; and, although they do not induce poisoning, still the result may be annoying and troublesome. They may almost invariably be dislodged and killed by the taking large draughts of salt and water.

Pieces of Glass, Coins, &c., may be inadvertently swallowed. Their treatment is named here, simply to dissuade the sufferer from the taking of purgatives, &c., to expel the foreign body; nor, on the other hand, should acid drinks be used which may render soluble, and so, possibly, poisonous, a coin or mass of metal otherwise inert. If the material in question have fairly passed into the stomach, nature will promote its exit in her own quiet way, and much more satisfactorily, too, than if the intestinal canal be tormented with drastic purgatives or unavailing emetic doses.

CHAPTER XI.

§ 1. *Suffocation: its Causes and their Treatment.*

SUFFOCATION, or, to use the medical term, asphyxia, is produced by those causes which impede or effectually prevent the entrance of air into the lungs. Thus it may be due to hanging, strangulation, or to drowning—these causes cutting off at once the air supply; or to breathing certain gases which do not support life, but which by hindering the access of pure air, induce a more tedious suffocation.

The blood is, under normal circumstances, sent from the large chamber on the right side of the heart to the lungs, to be there purified and freshly supplied with oxygen from the inspired air. If the supply of air be inadequate, the blood current, dark in colour and loaded with carbon, passes on through the left side of the heart and through the arteries to the brain and the body generally. It carries to these several tissues not life but poison, and as the air supply is more and more lessened, or even quite suppressed, each succeeding blood-wave is still less freed from carbon. The nervous system is narcotised by this impure blood, the heart lacking its usual stimulus ceases to act, and the processes both of circulation and respiration are stopped.

Suffocation may depend on—

I.—*Hanging or Strangulation.*

The element of danger and death in this condition is the mechanical occlusion of the windpipe, ensuring the shutting off of the entrance of atmospheric air. This may be gradual or immediate—usually the latter—

SUFFOCATION.

and insensibility and apparent death follow very rapidly.

By the speedy adoption of certain measures, life may, however, in a fair proportion of cases, be preserved.

The first requirement is to remove with all haste the rope or handkerchief which may have been tied round the neck. Cut the person down if he be found still hanging and place him gently on the ground, with the head somewhat raised above the level of the trunk. Remove the ligature from the neck, and after doing this any article of dress, handkerchief, shirt collar, &c., which may be pressing upon the neck or chest.

Artificial respiration (according to the rules given § 2 at the end of this section) may be put in practice.

Cold water may be dashed on the chest, and the surface directly afterwards should be rubbed dry with warm cloths. This same plan of friction may be extended, if there be sufficient help available, to the trunk and limbs, and should be carried out without intermission for some considerable time. Should there be much lividity about the face and chest, it will be wise to take away some blood. This may be done by an unskilled person easily, if he immerses one hand of the patient in warm water, and cuts through with a sharp knife or a razor some of the prominent veins on the back of the hand. The bleeding may be stopped by pressure with the finger. Or, again, leeches may be applied to the temples, twenty or thirty in number.

In all these instances of suspended animation, it is of especial importance that no time should be lost in a search for further or for more reliable assistance. The person first on the spot must carry out the above directions to the best of his ability and without delay.

II.—*Drowning.*

The actual condition is here due to the same cause as in death by hanging—the non-entrance of air into the lungs. If repeated attempts at breathing be made while the patient is in the water, air will escape from the chest, and water may pass into the air-passages, but this intrusion of water is no necessary condition of drowning.

Hence no attempts need be made, as our forefathers taught, to remove the water from the chest, by rolling the body face downwards on a barrel, &c.

The body should be taken to shelter, or to some room not too warm, so soon as it is removed from the water; the clothes removed as quickly as possible, and the surface dried with warm cloths; then at once artificial respiration (see § 2, at the end of this section) should be instituted.

The measure, however, of most apparent value, judging from recorded cases, in restoring the apparently dead from drowning, would seem to have been the steady and long-continued employment of friction of the whole surface of the body. Relays of attendants should be provided, and at regular intervals the changes of alternate sets should be made. Perseverance is imperative: in one most unpromising case (Dr. Douglas's) the time occupied was no less than eight hours and a half.

III.—*Breathing of Foul Air, Gases which cannot support Respiration, &c.*

Carbonic acid gas evolved from the burning of charcoal in rooms not provided with a chimney, or manufactured in the process of fermentation in breweries, or as existing in deep wells, excavations, &c., may be named as one of the compounds which may induce stifling or suffocation and death. Sulphuretted hydrogen, as generated by the decomposition of organic bodies, night-soil, &c., is equally operative in bringing on such symptoms.

The first point to be attended to is the removal of the sufferer, not only from the noxious atmosphere which he has been inhaling, but also to as pure an air as can be had. Expose him, therefore, to a free current of air outside the house, if the weather be fit, and dash cold water upon the face and chest; then have artificial respiration, if there be absolute arrest of breathing movements, employed, and for some time. Friction of the general surface may be combined with these measures, and, so soon as the patient can swallow, some hot coffee or brandy and water may be administered.

The probabilities of recovery are greater in this form of suffocation than either in cases of hanging or drowning. The arrest of the circulation is not always complete, and, though insensibility may remain for a time (simulating the effects of a dose of narcotic poison), yet in most cases of comparatively short exposure, recovery may be hoped for.

The workmen employed in emptying closed vaults, cellars, &c., in cleaning out the vats of brewhouses, or in any such work, need much to be cautioned about the risks they run. If one should fall insensible in the vault or vat, he must be removed at once by some mechanical means, if possible by a pole, rope, &c.; but if this fail, some second person should go in to rescue him, having, however, first taken the precaution to have a rope tied round him, so that the bystanders may so withdraw him and his burden, if he should in his turn be overcome by the foul air.

Whenever there is a fire in a stove or fireplace or on the ground, there should always be a chimney or flue for the free exit of the products of combustion. Not only is the air of a room rapidly spoiled by a fire which burns without a chimney, but it is speedily loaded with noxious fumes — rarely fatal, however, except to those who may have slept for hours in some such room, and when asleep have inspired the stupefying and poisonous gas.

In a minor degree yet of the same kind are the results perceived by those who have been breathing the air of some crowded theatre or public place, and so inspiring into their lungs air which has been thoroughly spoiled by the repeated respirations of many persons. Headache, drowsiness, faintness, and even stupor have their causes in this want of proper air for respiration. In children exposed to the influence of an impure atmosphere, sickness will very readily come on. Hence the golden rule, that no apartment is fit for continuous human habitation which does not allow of free ingress of fresh and egress of spoiled air, or which has not, if these conditions be unfulfilled, a very much larger cubic capacity than that required for the number of people present.

The smallest cubic space for each adult should be—

> In bedroom . . 300 cubic feet.
> In sitting-room, 400 ,,

§ 2. *Directions for Restoring the apparently Dead.*

As embodying in short space, and in terse and clear language, the most approved methods of resuscitation in those apparently dead from any form of asphyxia, the official copies of the Rules issued by the "Royal Humane Society," combined with those of the "Royal Life-boat Institution," have been reprinted in the following pages:—

SUFFOCATION.

I.—*Preliminary Rules.*

In cases of apparent death, either from drowning or other suffocation, send immediately for medical assistance, blankets, and dry clothing, but proceed to treat the patient *instantly* on the spot, in the open air, with the face downward, whether on shore or afloat; exposing the face, neck, and chest to the wind, except in severe weather, and removing all tight clothing from the neck and chest, especially the braces.

The points to be aimed at are—first and *immediately*, the *restoration of breathing;* and secondly, after breathing is restored, the *promotion of warmth and circulation.*

The efforts to *restore breathing* must be commenced immediately and energetically, and persevered in for one or two hours, or until a medical man has pronounced that life is extinct.

Efforts to promote *warmth and circulation*, beyond removing the wet clothes and drying the skin, must not be made until the first appearance of natural breathing. For if circulation of the blood be induced before breathing has recommenced, the restoration to life will be endangered.

II. — *Treatment to Restore Breathing, according to Dr. Marshall Hall's method.*

1. TO CLEAR THE THROAT,—

Place the patient on the floor or ground with the face downwards, and one of the arms under the forehead, in which position all fluids will more readily escape by the mouth, and the tongue itself will fall forward, leaving the entrance into the windpipe free. Assist this operation by wiping and cleansing the mouth.

If satisfactory breathing commences, use the treatment described below to promote

SUFFOCATION. 173

warmth. If there be only slight breathing —or no breathing—or if the breathing fail, then—

2. TO EXCITE BREATHING,—

Turn the patient well and instantly on the side, supporting the head, and excite the nostrils with snuff, hartshorn, and smelling salts, or tickle the throat with a feather, &c., if they are at hand. Rub the chest and face warm, and dash cold water, or cold and hot water alternately, on them.

If there be no success, lose not a moment, but instantly—

3. TO IMITATE BREATHING,—

Replace the patient on the face, raising and supporting the chest well on a folded coat or other article of dress.

Turn the body very gently on the side and a little beyond, and then briskly on the face, back again; repeating these measures

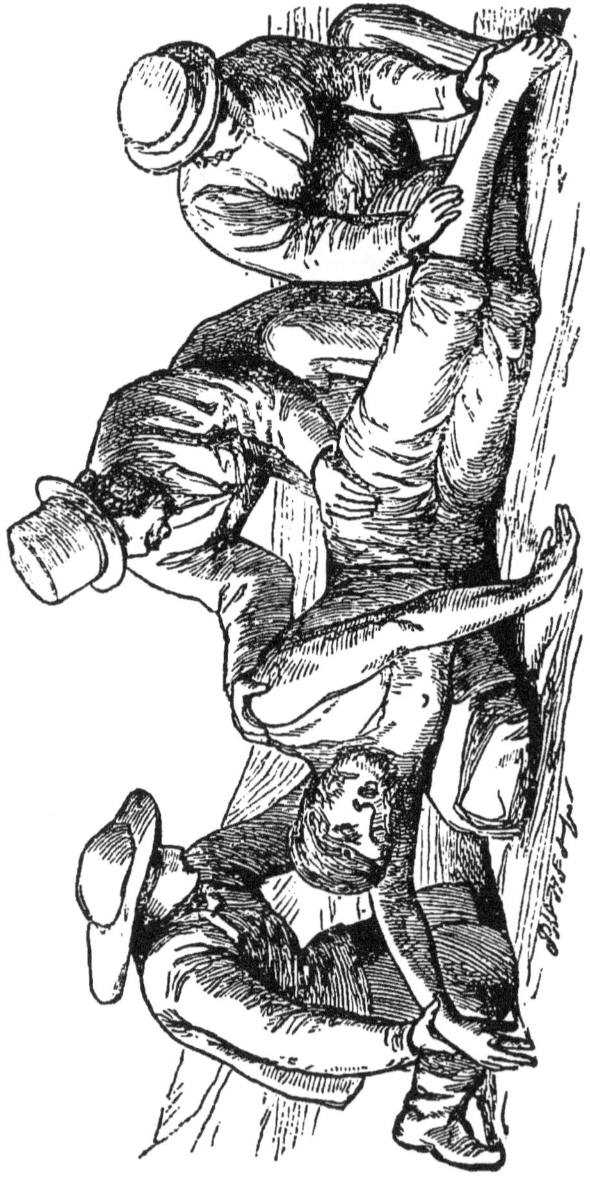

174 FIRST HELP IN ACCIDENTS.

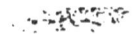

Fig. 28. Inspiration.

SUFFOCATION. 175

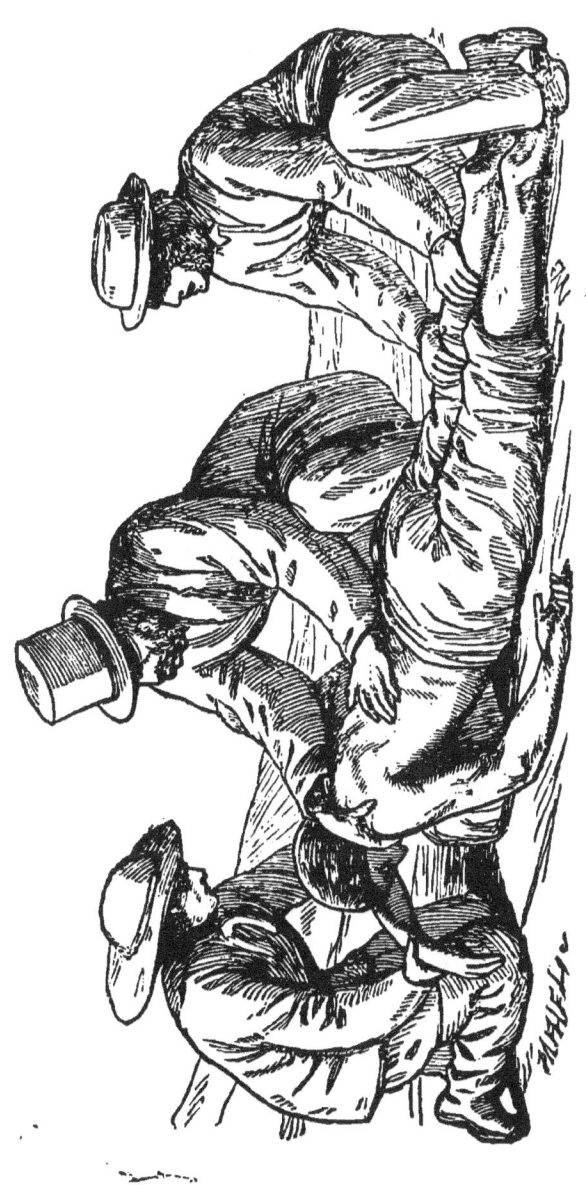

Fig. 29. Expiration.

cautiously, efficiently, and perseveringly about fifteen times in the minute, or once every four or five seconds, occasionally varying the side.

By placing the patient on the chest, the weight of the body forces the air out; when turned on the side, this pressure is removed, and air enters the chest.

The foregoing two illustrations (figs. 28 and 29) show the position of the body during the employment of Dr. Marshall Hall's method of inducing respiration.

On each occasion that the body is replaced on the face, make uniform but efficient pressure with brisk movement, on the back between and below the shoulder-blades or bones on each side, removing the pressure immediately before turning the body on the side.

During the whole of the operations let one person attend solely to the movements of the head, and of the arm placed under it.

The result is Respiration or Natural Breathing; and if not too late, Life.

Whilst the above operations are being proceeded with, dry the hands and feet; and as soon as dry clothing or blankets can be procured, strip the body and cover, or gradually reclothe it, but taking care not to interfere with the efforts to restore breathing.

III.—*Treatment to restore Breathing, according to Dr. Silvester's method.*

Instead of these proceedings, or should these efforts not prove successful in the course of from two to five minutes, proceed to imitate breathing by Dr. Silvester's method, as follows:—

Patient's position.

Place the patient on the back on a flat surface, inclined a little upwards from the feet; raise and support the head and shoulders on a small firm cushion or folded article of dress placed under the shoulder-blades.

2. *To effect a free entrance of air into the windpipe.*

Cleanse the mouth and nostrils, draw forward the patient's tongue, and keep it projecting beyond the lips: an elastic band over the tongue and under the chin will answer this purpose, or a piece of string or tape may be tied round them, or by raising the lower jaw, the teeth may be made to retain the tongue in that position. Remove all tight clothing from about the neck and chest, especially the braces.

3. *To imitate the movements of Breathing.*

Standing at the patient's head, grasp the arms just above the elbows, and draw the arms gently and steadily upwards above the head, and *keep them stretched* upwards for two seconds. (*By this means air is drawn into the lungs.*) Then turn down the patient's arms, and press them gently and firmly for two seconds against the sides of the chest. (See engravings 30 and 31, pp. 180, 181.) (*By this means air is pressed out of the lungs.* Pressure on the breastbone will aid this.)

Repeat these measures alternately, deliberately, and perseveringly, about fifteen times in a minute, until a spontaneous effort to respire is perceived, immediately upon which cease to imitate the movements of breathing, and proceed to *induce circulation and warmth.*

Should a warm bath be procurable, the body may be placed in it up to the neck, continuing to imitate the movements of breathing. Raise the body in twenty seconds in a sitting position, and dash cold water against the chest and face, and pass ammonia under the nose. The patient should not be kept in the warm bath longer than five or six minutes.

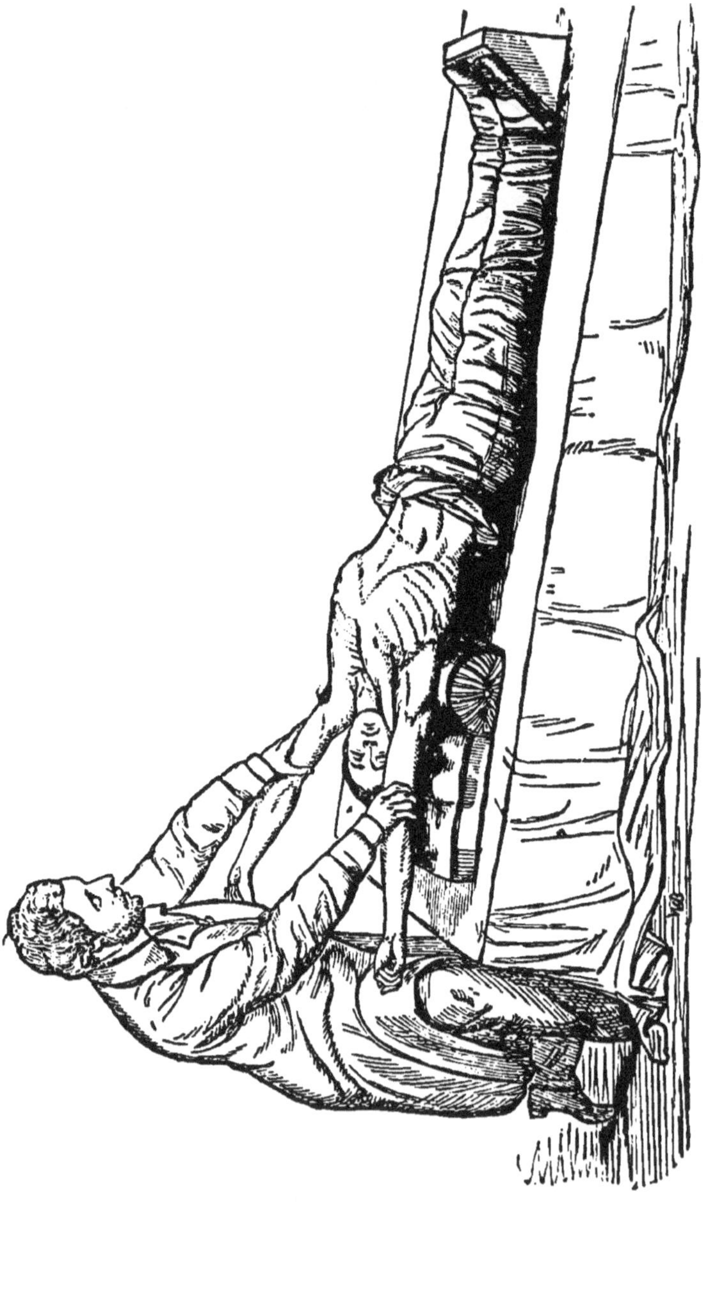

180   FIRST HELP IN ACCIDENTS.

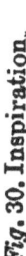

Fig. 30. Inspiration.

SUFFOCATION.

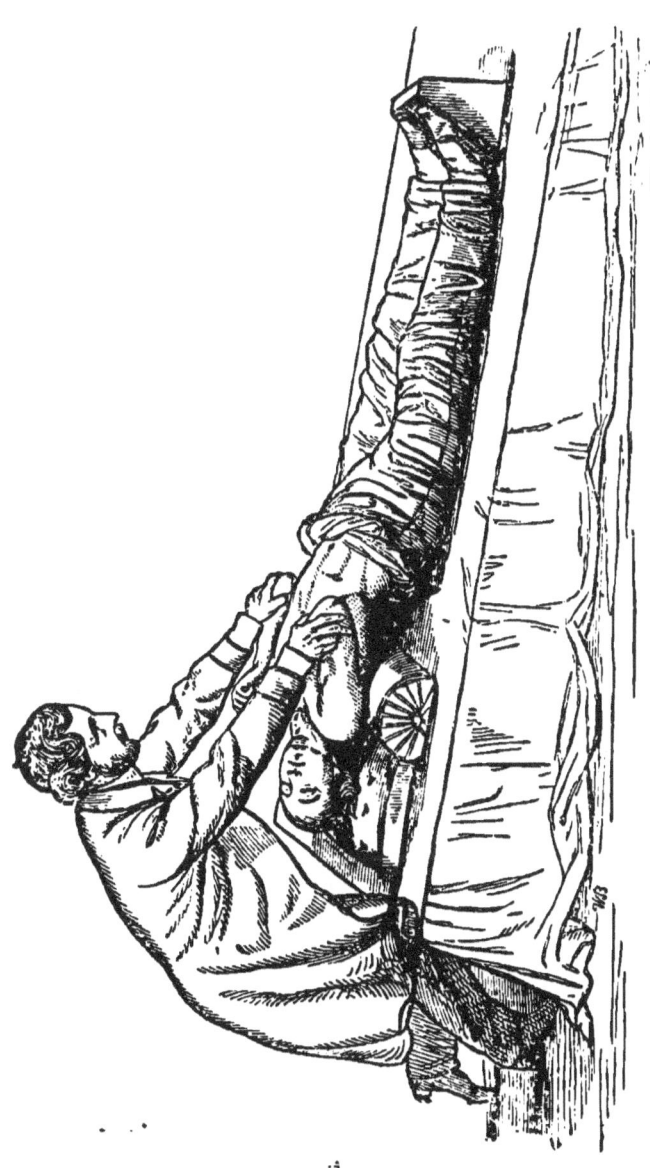

Fig. 31. Expiration.

4. *To excite Inspiration.*

During the employment of the above method excite the nostrils with snuff or smelling-salts, or tickle the throat with a feather. Rub the chest and face briskly, and dash cold and hot water alternately on them.

The above directions are chiefly Dr. H. R. Silvester's method of restoring the apparently dead or drowned, and have been approved by the Royal Medical and Chirurgical Society.*

IV.—*Treatment after Natural Breathing has been Restored.*

1. *To promote Warmth and Circulation,*

Wrap the patient in dry blankets, commence rubbing the limbs upwards, with

---

* The author would wish here to acknowledge the courtesy of the Secretary of the Royal Humane Society, who has placed at his disposal the woodcuts of figures 30 and 31.

firm grasping pressure and energy, using handkerchiefs, flannels, &c. (*By this measure the blood is propelled along the veins towards the heart.*)

The friction must be continued under the blanket or over the dry clothing.

Promote the warmth of the body by the application of hot flannels, bottles, or bladders of hot water, heated bricks, &c., to the pit of the stomach, the arm-pits, between the thighs, and to the soles of the feet. Warm clothing may generally be obtained from bystanders.

2. If the patient has been carried to a house after respiration has been restored, be careful to let the air play freely about the room.

3. On the restoration of life, when the power of swallowing has returned, a teaspoonful of warm water, small quantities of wine, warm brandy and water, or coffee, should be administered. The patient should be kept in bed, and a disposition to sleep

encouraged. During reaction, large mustard plasters to the chest below the shoulders will greatly relieve the distressed breathing.

V.—*General Observations.*

The above treatment should be persevered in for some hours, as it is an erroneous opinion that persons are irrecoverable because life does not soon make its appearance, persons having been restored after persevering for many hours.

VI.—*Appearances which generally indicate Death.*

Breathing and the heart's action cease entirely; the eyelids are generally half closed; the pupils dilated; the jaws clenched; the fingers semi-contracted; the tongue approaches to the under edges of the lips, and these, as well as the nostrils, are covered with a frothy mucus. Coldness and pallor of surface increase.

VII.—*Cautions.*

1. Prevent unnecessary crowding of persons round the body, especially if in an apartment.

2. Avoid rough usage, and do not allow the body to remain on the back unless the tongue is secured.

3. Under no circumstances hold the body up by the feet.

4. On no account place the body in a warm bath, unless under medical direction, and even then it should only be employed as a momentary excitant.

CHAPTER XII.

OF THE SIGNS OF REAL DEATH.

IT is needless to insist on the importance of being able to distinguish between apparent and real death. Profound faintness (syncope) or asphyxia, resulting in the first instance on severe physical injuries, or on overpowering mental emotion; in the second condition on prolonged submersion, suspension, or exposure to non-respirable vapours, may either of them so far interfere with the processes of circulation and respiration as to raise in the mind of a bystander the idea that the person is really dead. Under these conditions death, however, is only simulated : the functions of the body have reached their lowest degree of action;

there is infrequent and hardly perceptible respiration; the heart still continues to circulate blood, but its beat is feeble, and the arterial or pulse-wave can hardly be distinguished; the surface of the body will be cold and clammy, and ordinary stimuli have no effect. There is, however, no chemical alteration in the tissues of the body.

Even a stage further than this may the suspension of the external manifestations of life be carried, and yet the person cannot be said to be dead; thus recovery has been known to occur in cases of drowning, where neither pulse nor respiration could be decidedly said to exist, and the frictions employed in the promotion of artificial respiration, &c., have been continued for hours before further signs of life declared their existence. Such instances, however, are to a degree exceptional, and their possible occurrence would simply point out the duty of continuing attempts at resuscitation, even in the absence for some hours of any symptoms of life.

When death has really occurred there usually comes on, even with great rapidity, pallor of the external surface; the temperature of the body sinks with more or less rapidity, according to the warmth of the surrounding atmosphere; the eye loses some of its lustre, and the pupils are usually dilated; respiration and circulation have ceased; within a few hours the limbs become rigid and fixed in their positions, and later on the textures show evidence of chemical decay; putrefaction commences, and the first external signs of this are specially to be found in the swelling and change of colour of the abdominal surface. The eyes later on are flat and sunken, and the body as a whole undergoes well marked putrefactive changes.

The practical points, however, are these:—

If the heart-beat cannot be detected by the

ear applied close to the left side of the chest, near to the left nipple, and pulsation have ceased in the arteries of the neck and arm; if the chest remains thoroughly motionless, and the rising and falling of the ribs can no longer even in small degree be observed, while a mirror put before the mouth has no dimness on its surface from moisture, then the bystander will be justified in concluding that death has occurred.

But as a spark of vitality may still remain, if the death seem to have followed on drowning or hanging, it will be well that the rules laid down in a preceding chapter for the restoration of persons so situated should be put in practice, and carried out for some considerable time.

"Lateat scintillula forsan."

CHAPTER XIII.

OF THE MEANS TO BE EMPLOYED IN THE TRANSPORT OF INJURED PERSONS AND INVALIDS.

IN all cases of accident or illness, the transport of the sufferer must only be decided on after the immediate and first assistance has been afforded in local dressings or remedial measures, and when those in charge are well satisfied that the proposed removal will not prove injurious. The latter consideration will often need to be dismissed from the mind under conditions of urgency and haste, but where there is a choice of action full weight should be given to the demands of each special case before removal to a greater or less distance be attempted.

§ 1. *Transport without special means for the purpose.*

If the sufferer from wound received in the battle-field or from accidental injury have escaped injury in his lower limbs, it may be quite possible for him in slight cases, after the first shock of the damage has passed by, to walk at least some short distance. For this purpose he will need the assistance of one person, and may support himself by the arm of his attendant, either leaning his weight upon it, or having the companion's arm thrown around his back or shoulders; or the sufferer may be taken bodily on the back of a strong and willing comrade. The help of two persons may be needed to allow the patient to walk with comfort; they can afford support by passing the arms round the back, &c.

In cases where the number of injured

persons is large, or that of assistants very limited, the sufferers, even those with wounds on the lower limbs, might be enabled to reach a place of shelter by means of crutches. Figure 32 shows a man walking on crutches which, by

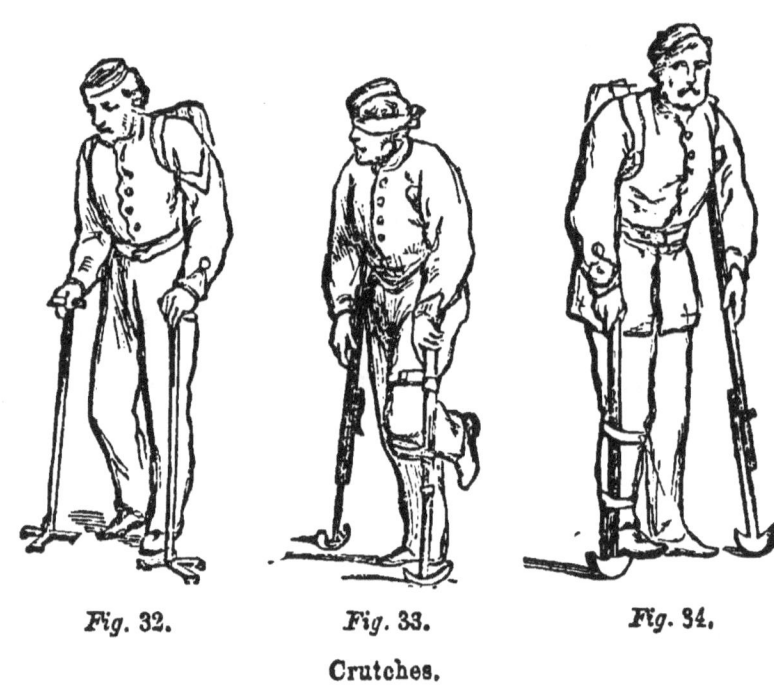

Fig. 32.   *Fig. 33.*   *Fig. 34.*

Crutches.

means of cross-pieces at the lower end, do not sink in soft ground. Figures 33 and 34 represent persons on crutches (proposed by Dr. Esmarch) which can be adjusted to any length of limbs; the limb is attached to the crutch by a strap; the foot rests either upon an iron support projecting towards the inside at the bottom of the crutch, or the knee rests upon a knee-splint projecting from the crutch at the height of the knee.

Walking must not be allowed to the wounded man, if he have had loss of consciousness, with severe injury of the head, or if he have had penetrating wound of the chest, or excessive loss of blood.

It may happen that the injury is such that the sufferer cannot walk from damage to his lower limbs, or from the severity of the wound. In this case he must be carried, and if the distance be but short, and the patient light and slim, it will be possible that *one* attendant may carry him. This is best managed by taking the patient in a sitting posture in his arms, the right arm being placed under the thighs, clasping them well together, while the left arm is thrown round the trunk under the shoulders, the patient meanwhile having his right arm thrown round the neck of the assistant. But if the sufferer is to be carried a longer distance by *one* man, the position in the accompanying figure 35 is recommended, as least fatiguing to the bearer. The sufferer is attached by two cross-belts to the back of his bearer.

If *two* persons are available (and for a heavy man, they must be had), the patient may still be carried in the sitting posture: the attendants, one on each side, clasping their right hands beneath the thighs, and with the left hands supporting the back, may so move him with fair ease. The patient may steady and support himself by grasping with his hands the shoulders of his bearers. Or, again, the attendants

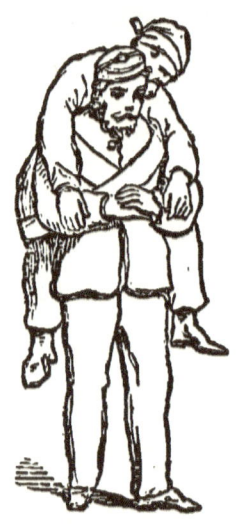

Fig. 35. Carrying.

walking sideways may carry more firmly by placing both hands each one on his own side, beneath the thighs of the supported person, while the injured man supports his trunk by grasping with his own hands the shoulders of the bearers as before. The carriers may become tired, or it may seem well to move the patient while he remains in a horizontal position, and then this plan may be adopted. One bearer lifting the head and shoulders may support the weight of the upper part of the trunk by placing his arms well under the armpits of the sufferer; the other helper may take charge of the lower limbs, so leaving the centre without direct support.

There is another mode of carrying a sufferer, whose injuries are not very serious, for a long distance. The patient sits upon a staff or musket, which is carried by two men as in the accompanying figure 36, and slings his arms around theirs. Additional aid should, if possible, be had in any case where there may have been severe injury to the lower limbs, so that the

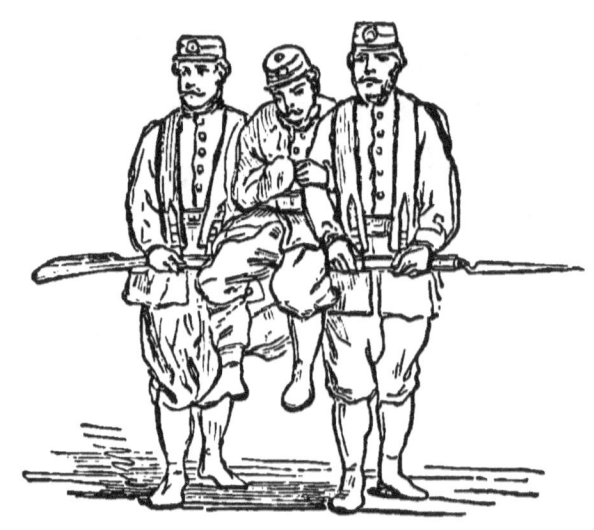

Fig. 36. Musket-Litter.

damaged part may receive the sole attention of one person, and so be preserved from shaking or displacement.

It will frequently happen that this mode of transport is the only one available. If it should appear from the description to be inconvenient or awkward, there are yet certain positive advantages inseparable from the employment of a human litter at once intelligent and sympathizing.

2. *Transport by Litters.*

There are two kinds of litters—those which are extempore, made on the spot from any available materials, and those which have been constructed for this express purpose.

Those only which allow of ready construction, and can be put together by any intelligent person, will have an especial notice. The second kind have by various inventors been brought to great perfection, but their description does not fall within the scope of this little work.

A litter should be strong, comfortable, —not liable to change its form or the arrangement of its separate parts, and must be of such a size and shape that the sufferer can obtain full rest for his person.

In the accidents occurring in everyday life, it will sometimes be sufficient for the removal of an injured person, to make use of a simple frame made of four pieces of wood, just so long that tied together at the corners they constitute a flat surface, on which the patient may sit easily and firmly. The projecting ends of the poles then afford good hand-hold to two bearers, and across the poles to support the weight may be twisted some twigs or small branches, or two or more cravat handkerchiefs may be tied across for the same purpose.

Or, again, for the purpose of transport in the horizontal position, a hurdle or sheep-tray may be employed. A shutter taken from a shop window, or, in case of need, a door lifted off its hinges, will also be available. Pieces of wood, too, of the required length, may be fastened together by some hasty appliances, twisted round and round, for instance, with a cart-rope, to hold them firm in the necessary position.

If any of these appliances be used, the upper surface should be well packed, for the greater comfort of the invalid, with some small rolls of straw, great coats, rugs, &c., or some clothes borrowed from the bystanders.

A very satisfactory litter, if a long transit be imperative, may be constructed by four poles — two eight feet long, two about four feet long. The two long

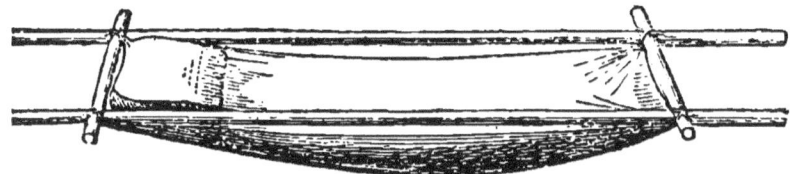

Fig. 37. Blanket-Litter.

poles, placed parallel with each other at a distance of about three feet, should be intersected by the two shorter poles, so as to leave an open space between the four poles measuring about six feet by three feet. Having tied the poles firmly together where they cross one another, a blanket should be fastened securely to them, so as to make the whole resemble the frame and sacking of a bedstead. (See fig. 37.) Upon this blanket the patient may be placed, and then the projecting ends of the poles may be carried, according to circumstances, by two or by four assistants.

If a mattress be at hand, strongly

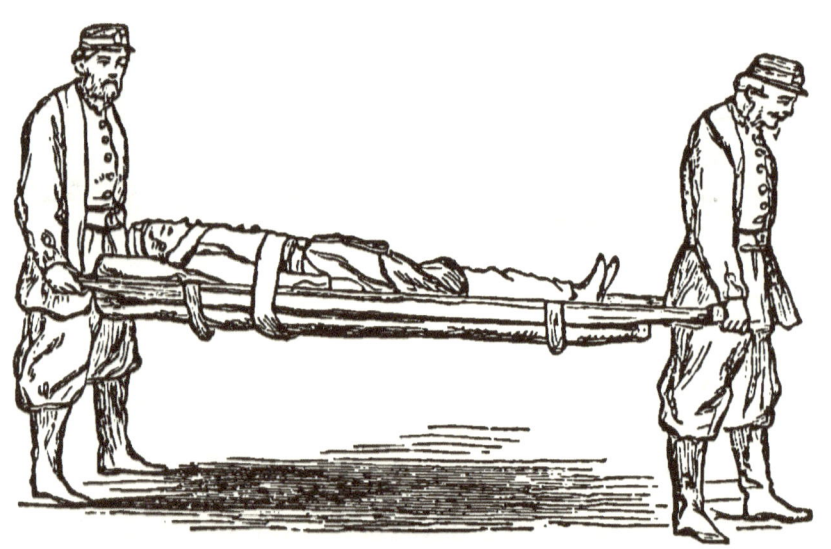

Fig. 38. Mattress-Litter.

made either of hair or of straw, this may be used as a litter by putting a loop of rope through each corner, so that by these loops the litter may be conveniently carried. (See fig. 38.)

On military service, good temporary litters may be made from muskets, a knapsack or two, and some cravat bandages or knapsack straps.

If the injured man be able to sit up, two muskets will be sufficient. These should be so placed parallel to one another, that upon, or rather between them, a knapsack may be fastened as a seat, by passing the straps round the barrel and lock of the musket on each side. A cravat or handkerchief will aid in making the whole arrangement thoroughly firm, if it be tied firmly round one corner of the knapsack, and then brought across beneath the framework, to meet another handkerchief which has already been fastened to the opposite corner.

Should it, however, be necessary to remove the wounded man in a horizontal position, four muskets will be required. They must be arranged as the poles are in the pole and blanket-litter named above (see fig. 37), and the vacant space between the muskets, first well fastened together at their corners by straps or cravats, may then be filled up by some knapsacks, four or more, as may be required, closely bound to one another, and to the musket framework by straps and handkerchiefs. Upon these knapsacks so arranged, some cloaks or coats may be thrown, so as to make a softer reclining-place for the sufferer.

Unless rapidity of movement be essential, it will be well that, before the invalid is fairly taken *en route,* he should be allowed to test the litter on which he is to recline, both with regard to the strength of the framework and the packing of the coverings. Much care should be given to the placing of the head in a slightly raised position, to the firm fixing of any fractured or dislocated limb, and to the due retention of any dressings which may have been applied to the injured part.

Both in lifting the litter, and in marching onwards with their burden, the bearers on each side must act together. The pace should be equal, and the step kept time to time, or the litter will be so much jarred by any irregular movement as to cause even serious annoyance to the patient.

§ 3. *Transport by Vehicles.*

As with litters for transport, so with vehicles. One kind are specially constructed with this end in view, and so are supplied to armies in the field—of these, no further mention will be made in these pages. Those, however, with which we have to deal, are vehicles originally made for other purposes, employed for demands of agriculture or daily transit, and which, yet with some trifling modifications, may be made available for the satisfactory transport of the wounded or the sick.

It is essential that the carriage selected for this purpose should be firm and strong. If the choice be afforded, a four-wheeled carriage should be preferred to one with two wheels, and so, too, one with springs is better than one which has the body fixed directly and firmly upon the axletree. Little needs to be said about the use of all those light vehicles which are built for domestic convenience and are easily moved from place to place.

The seats already existing in the interior of such carriages are at once available for wounded men who are able to keep the sitting posture; and, provided that there be sufficient length from end to end of the vehicle, one or more may be accommodated in the reclining position upon straw mattresses, rugs, &c.

Slightly wounded persons may also be placed in a sitting posture on two chairs or two carriage seats. The legs are placed upon a board covered with a sack filled

TRANSPORT OF INJURED PERSONS. 205

with hay or straw. The board may be placed upon the front and back seat of a railway carriage. (See fig. 39.)

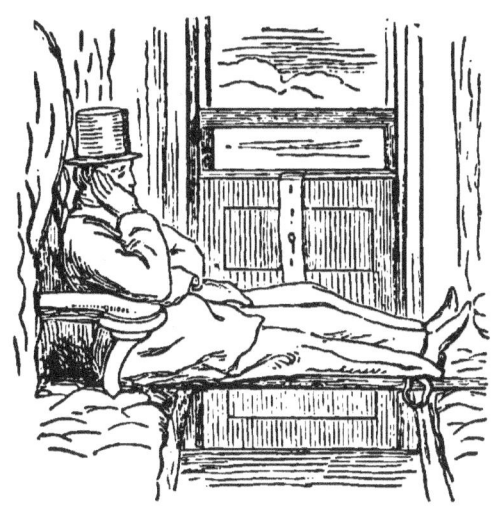

Fig. 39. Transport in a Railway Carriage.

Another plan of transporting more severely injured persons in luggage vans or carts is illustrated by figure 40.

In order to prevent severely wounded persons suffering from the shaking of the vehicles, they might be transported in luggage vans, or in large carts, in the manner represented by figure 41, suspended litter.

Figures 42, 43, and 44 represent various

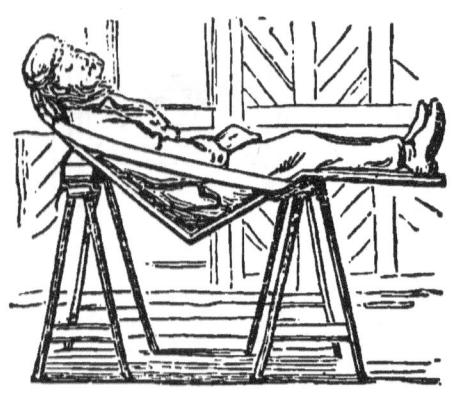

Fig. 40. Transport in Luggage Carriages and Cart.

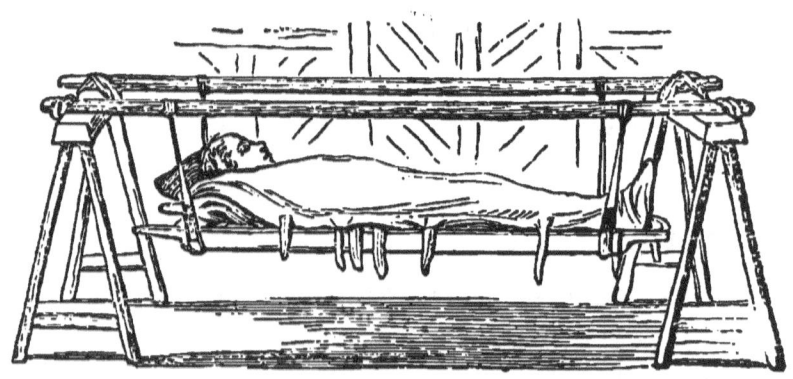

Fig. 41. Suspended Litter.

kinds of two-wheeled transport carts, built by Messrs. Fischer & Co., in Heidelberg, the well-known manufacturers of surgical

TRANSPORT OF INJURED PERSONS. 207

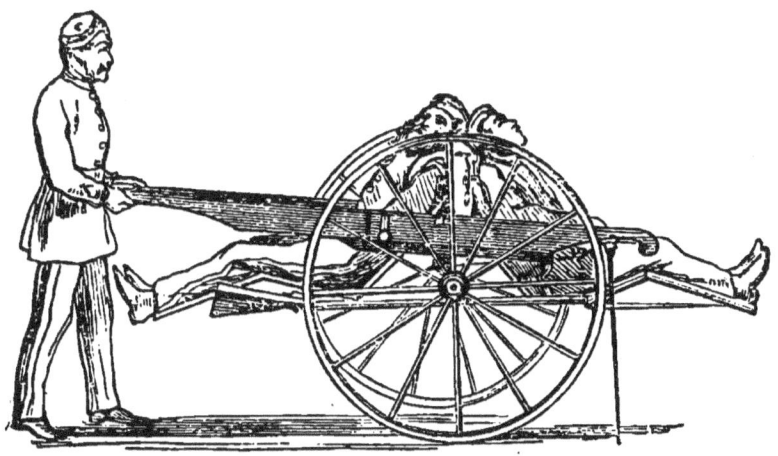

Fig. 42. Two-Wheeled Transport Cart.

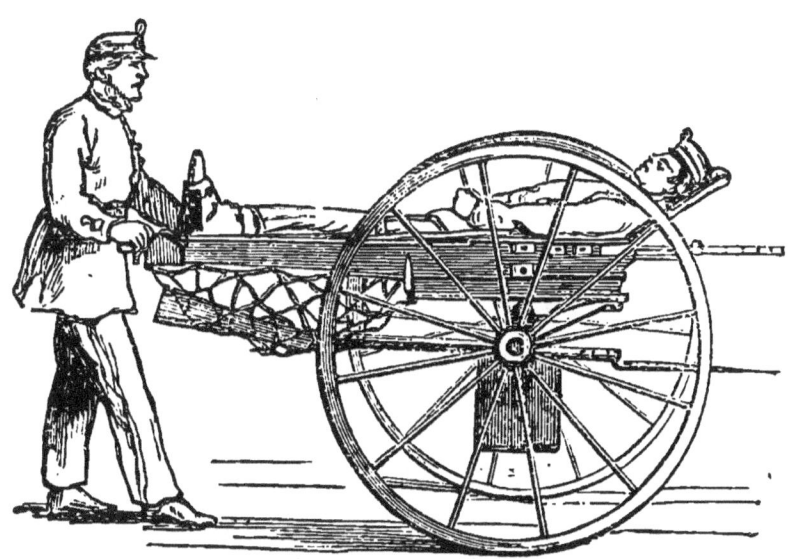

Fig. 43. Two-Wheeled Transport Cart.

and hygienic apparatus. Any cart might be easily arranged for the same purpose, and according to a similar plan. Either a

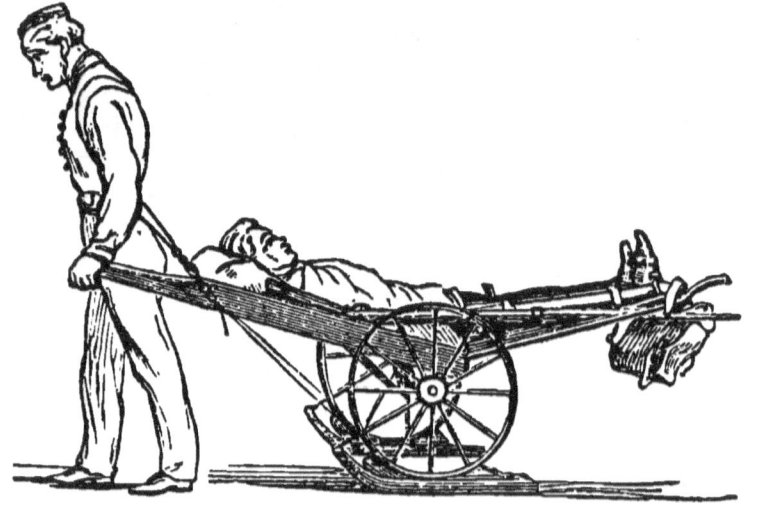

Fig. 44. Two-Wheeled Sledge Litter.

litter, arranged for a lying or a sitting position, may be laid upon it, or two arm-chairs be suspended on it, for carrying one or two sufferers. For transport on snow, muddy or hilly ground, the wheels may be put on sledges (fig. 44), and such a litter may be either wheeled, carried, or used as a sledge.

To make an ordinary field-cart available

for the removal of wounded men, ropes must be carried backwards and forwards from one side to the other of the upper ledge of the framework, and well fastened by knots or twisting to the wooden frame, so as to form an elastic, or at least a movable floor, upon which straw in long bundles, branches of trees, rugs, &c., may be laid so as to form a hammock swinging freely from side to side of the cart; upon this one or two men may easily be placed. The ropes must be drawn so tight that when the mattress and men are placed upon them, they shall still hang at some little distance from the wooden bottom of the vehicle. Seats may in the same way be arranged at each end to accommodate two men who are able to sit up. Knapsacks, luggage, &c., may be placed beneath the extemporized bed. The sun, rain, or wind may be kept from the occupants by bending some hoops or sticks archwise over them, fastening the ends to the cart body, and over these frames throwing a cloth or cloak.

The driving must be very slow as a rule; every shock or violent movement should be studiously avoided, and all moving to and from the carriages should be managed in the most gentle manner, either by the use of hand litters, or by the arms of assistants used to the same end. Wounds and fractures imply in the vast majority of cases very considerable suffering; it would be cruelty itself to add to this the pain of ill-regulated means of removal from place to place.

The slow pace at which travelling is possible, and the distances to be traversed, make some provision for the nourishment of the wounded to be imperative. Thirst, very commonly complained of, must be met by supplies of cold water. Tea or coffee with soups may be also given, but meat and stimulants are on such a journey best avoided; the occurrence of faintness may make the use of the latter compounds advisable, but even then they should be but sparingly given.

§ 4. *Transport upon Animals.*

After engagements in which cavalry may have been actively employed, horses may with advantage be employed to remove wounded soldiers as quickly as possible from the field. The soldier may lead a horse upon the saddle of which he has placed a wounded comrade, or seated himself on the animal's back he may support the patient seated in some straw or a folded rug in front of him, and hold the wounded man from falling by his right arm passed round the chest. The left arm will be occupied by the bridle.

A chair or seat may be slung on each side of a quiet horse, and thus two wounded soldiers able to sit up may be conveyed. Or in some conditions, if the reclining posture be required, the mattress upon which the patient lies may be suspended from the harness of two horses, one horse being placed on each side. To each horse an attendant should be assigned for the more perfect security of the patient so conveyed.

CHAPTER XIV.

HYGIENIC RULES FOR WALKING AND FOR MARCHES.—ACCIDENTS WHICH MAY HAPPEN TO SOLDIERS ON MARCH, ETC.

THE following directions may be of service to the civilian who undertakes from necessity or from choice a long and fatiguing walk—to the soldier on march, and to the officers who may have charge of detachments for special purposes and forced journeys.

1. Clothing should be loosely fitting throughout; no stiff or tight neckcloths; no ligatures tied more or less tightly round the limbs. Woollen materials are far the best for the outer garments; flannel for those worn next the skin.

2. The colour of the outer dress, if choice

can be allowed, should be light, white or some shade of grey—especially must this rule be followed where the sun has much power. A black dress is of all the most unpleasant for a long walk.

3. The head should be sheltered by a cap or felt hat—soft, flexible, and perforated with holes, so that air has ready access to the surface of the head. A peak for the warding off sun rays from the eyes, and a hood to protect the back of the head and the neck, will both be of some advantage. In tropical climates a white cover over all would be very advantageous.

4. The feet should be clothed with light worsted socks; and shoes or boots should be worn which are not too tight for the foot, and which are so made by having the inside edge of the front part of each boot parallel to that of its fellow, that the toes are not cramped together in a cone or wedge-shaped front. The form of each sole ought to correspond exactly with the

natural form of the foot-sole. Above all let the heels be no thicker than the rest of the sole. A more abominable phrase than the term "military heels" was never introduced. The height is slightly increased to the detriment of the soldier in every other particular.

Blisters and sore feet may well happen after a long march: the former are best treated by passing a single thread of worsted from side to side through each blister, and leaving it for a day undisturbed. Sore feet are much relieved by tepid bathing, having first dissolved in the water a small quantity of common salt or alum.

5. If weight must be carried, the bundle should be so placed between the shoulders that it rests there without muscular exertion, and the framework of the knapsack should take its support by light iron rods upon the bony framework of the pelvis, and not be hung by straps which pass across the chest. A clean shirt, some soap, a pair of

clean socks, and a light waterproof overcoat, will form the greater part of the package necessary for a pedestrian tourist.

6. If the arrangement be at all feasible, some daily practice should be had in walking distances preparatory to a long journey, each day increasing the ground passed over, so that the pedestrian may not enter on his task quite unused to the exercise.

7. The time occupied in walking should be, if possible, so divided that some rest may be obtained in the middle of the day, and so while the heat is greatest. Food should be plain, nutritious, and not too watery or bulky: the pemmican or prepared meat of the North-American Indian is probably the best type of portable food for a pedestrian.

The accidents which most probably will happen to soldiers on a march are—

Faintness: this may be slight, or may pass on to positive unconsciousness—the patient turns pale, would fall if no support be given, and may have muscular tremors, or even threatening of convulsions.

The treatment will consist in placing the patient flat on the ground, dashing cold water over him, and administering some stimulant.

Causes which aggravate or induce the tendency to this condition, are to be found in carelessness about the taking of food, disturbance of the bowels, &c., and perhaps more especially in the marching with ranks very close, so that those men toward the centre have deficient supply of fresh air. Therefore, to guard against the possibility of this happening, in frequent instances the ranks should be opened out as much as possible; the position of the men changed occasionally from the centre to the outside files, and, if it be possible, an occasional rest, with the refreshment of some coffee or tea, should be arranged.

Exhaustion may be spoken of as the

sequel of severe faintness, or as occurring from much exertion, in the instance of some man who is not physically capable of undergoing fatigue; the sufferer becomes partially faint, dizzy, and confused; struggles for a time to keep up with his comrades, and blindly stumbles on ultimately to fall from sheer want of vigour.

Rest more or less prolonged in the horizontal position, food, and quiet, are necessary to the restoration of power.

Sunstroke or heat apoplexy has been already referred to. See Chapter VI., § 2, p. 87.

CHAPTER XV.

RÉSUMÉ OF DIRECTIONS FOR THE TREATMENT OF SEVERE ACCIDENTS OR INJURIES.

LET it be distinctly understood that the immediate treatment of any severely injured person has a positive influence, not only on the early stages of the progress to recovery, but also on the whole treatment; whether this be in the hands of a non-professional attendant, or it be possible to obtain the skilled services of some medical man with but little delay.

1. Make out as exact a history as may be done from patient or bystanders.

2. Place the patient in a suitable position on side in preference to placing him flat on his back. Remove clothing.

3. Cold water may be applied externally

and given also internally. Stimulants should be avoided except in cases urgently demanding their administration.

4. Do not bleed merely because an accident has happened.

5. Examine the patient gently and yet very carefully; very probably he will be lying on the ground, and if so make the first examination without raising him: it is a bad practice hastily to pick a man up when he is faint from shock, and may have severe injury to some part of the frame. If the ground be damp, let some coat or cloak be quickly drawn under the patient: then the dress must be loosened or removed, and this not by dragging it off the limbs, but by opening the seams, &c., with knife or scissors.

If there be *wound* incised or contused, wash it well with sponge or linen dipped in water, so as to arrest bleeding and remove foreign substances.

6. If there be bleeding to inconsiderable

amount, it may even be encouraged; but if there be some quantity of blood pouring away, the directions given at length in Chapter II., p. 33, must be strictly followed.

7. The wound whether incised, contused, or inflicted by rifle bullet must be treated in accordance with the rules given in Chapter III., p. 53. Immediate closure of the wound, if it be at all practicable, should be carried out by the means there recommended.

8. If it happen that there is *spraining* of some joint, the wounded part may at the moment be supported by putting on a bandage well wetted with cold water. If this bandage cannot conveniently be removed, it may be kept well wetted by pouring cold water upon it.

The patient may be in the house, and then thorough rest with constant irrigation, drop by drop, of cold water will usually be found preferable. (See Chapter I., § 2, and Chapter VII., p. 91.)

9. *Dislocation* of some joint may have

happened—rest must be insisted on, and until a surgeon can arrive, cold applications should be used to the injured part; the limb should be kept quiet either with bandaging or by position.

In the case of some few dislocations, an attempt at reduction may be made by a non-professional attendant if no skilled assistance can be had. For these and further directions see Chapter VII., p. 93.

10. If some bone have been *fractured* the injured part must be so moved that it assumes in a measure at least its normal appearance, and then retained in a fairly easy position. The transport of the patient must be managed with much care.

If the upper extremity or the collar-bone be fractured in any part, the limb must be fastened to the body by some cravat bandages, or by several turns of a roller so as to prevent jarring or shaking: a sling, too, in addition to the bandage will afford some support.

If there be fracture of the lower extremity, the patient should first be placed on some convenient level surface and the limb adjusted. As a temporary measure during transport, the injured part may be supported by fastening to it a large and soft pillow and cushion: the limb placed upon this may be retained in place by some turns of a roller embracing both cushion and limb.

Or, again, it will be quite possible and often best to make the sound limb the temporary splint for the other one. Interposing some thin pads between the knees and ankles, the operator may fasten both limbs together by two or more cravat bandages. In either case it is of importance to support the foot, and to prevent its turning either in an inward or outward direction. (See Chapter VIII., p. 103.)

1. No direct mention has been made of injuries to the eyes: foreign bodies (in military life grains of powder or fragments of percussion caps, and in civil life insects, grains of sand, &c.) are not infrequently jerked in between the eyelid and the globe of the eye itself.

The patient must not yield to the desire to rub his eye; but the bystander should draw down first the lower then the upper lid, and look for the offending fragment. It is often easy to remove it with the tip of the finger, or the corner of a handkerchief twisted into a point. A camel-hair pencil may be available.

While the manipulation is going on, the patient should look before him at some steady object.

Afterwards the eye must be closed with a pad of linen, and a light handkerchief be bound over this round the head.

12. For details of treatment of special injuries, so far as the space of this little

work has allowed of their consideration, reference must be made to the separate chapters. The more uncommon forms of accident, poisonings, &c., must also be sought for under their appropriate headings.

APPENDIX.

LIST OF ARTICLES for dressings, instruments, appliances for external use, and medicines recommended in the "First Help for Accidents," which might be kept in store in a household, or on board a vessel that does not carry a surgeon.

The figures refer to the pages on which the articles in question are named.

1. *Articles for Dressings.* (Must be kept dry and clean in a box.)

   Bandages, rollers, compresses, of various length and breadth (of calico or linen), 14, 54.
   Bladder, 21.
   Flannel, 10, 24, 25.
   Gutta Percha (strong, for splints), 112, 130.
   Gutta Percha (tissue), 10, 25.
   India-rubber Bag, 21.
   Linen, 11.
   Lint, 10.
   Oil-cloth, 22.
   Oil Silk, 10, 25.
   Pasteboard, 112.
   Plaster (adhesive), 11, 54, 55.

FIRST HELP IN ACCIDENTS. 227

Silk (sewing for ligatures), 51.
Splints, 13.
Sponges, 9.
Straps, 112.

2. *Instruments.* (Must be kept separate in a leather case, and cleaned after having been used.)
Caustic Holder. (See Caustics.)
Dressing Forceps, 19, 53.
Lancet, 19.
Scalpel, 19.
Scissors, 18.
Suture Needles, 19, 52, 54, 56, 57.
Syringe for Injections, holding one or two ounces.
Syringe for Clysters. (*Ex. gr.*, Higginson's Elastic Enema.)
Tenaculum, 18, 51.
Tourniquet, 18, 46.

3. *Appliances (medicinal and other) for External Use.* (Medicines to be kept in a separate box, in stoppered bottles, labelled.)
Acacia, Gum, 112.
Astringents, local, 70.
Arnica (lotion), 73.
Balsam, Friar's, 66, 108.
Calamine Ointment, 70, 79.
Camomile Flowers, 24.
Caustics (employed with a holder or a quill pen) :—
    Nitrate of silver, 157.
    Sulphate of copper (blue stone), 62.
Deodorizers : any one of the following suffices :—
    Chloride of Lime, 71.
    Chloride of Soda, 71.

Chloride of Zinc, 71.
Condy's Patent Fluid, 71.
Flour, 78.
Hops, 24.
Leeches, 28, 64.
Linseed Meal, 26.
Mustard, 27.
Oil, 78.
Resin Ointment, 78.
Starch, 78, 112.
Turpentine, 78.
Vinegar, 81.

4. *Medicines for Internal Use.* (Kept in a separate box, in stoppered bottles, labelled.)

Alkalies—soda, potash, magnesia, 149.

Emetics—
    Ipecacuanha Wine, 146.
    Mustard and water, 146.
    Salt and water, 146.
    Sulphate of Zinc (in 10-grain packets), 136, 146.

Stimulants—
    Brandy, 31.
    Coffee, 31.
    Tea, 31.

THE END

Fcap. 8vo. cloth, price 2s. 6d.

THE
HOME NURSE:

A MANUAL

FOR

THE SICK ROOM.

BY

ESTHER LE HARDY.

" There is much useful information in Miss Le Hardy's book."—*Lancet.*

" Extremely serviceable to all who have at any time to do with the chamber of sickness."—*Reader.*

LONDON:
ROBERT HARDWICKE, 192, PICCADILLY, W.

USEFUL WORKS

PUBLISHED BY

ROBERT HARDWICKE,

192, PICCADILLY, W.

Practical Physiology: a Manual of Health.
Being a Practical Guide to the Means of Securing Health and Life. Intended for the use of classes and general reading. By Dr. LANKESTER, F.R.S. Fifth Edition, Fcap. 8vo., illustrated, price 2s. 6d.

"It is copiously illustrated. There is not a school of any kind for males or females, rich or poor, in which the book might not be used as a text-book; indeed, it ought to be as common as an English Grammar. Few persons are capable of forming an idea of the increase of human happiness and material prosperity which would follow a more general appreciation of the laws of health."—*Lancet*.

Dr. Lankester on the Uses of Animals
In Relation to the Industry of Man. By EDWIN LANKESTER, M.D., F.R.S. A Course of Six Lectures delivered at the South Kensington Museum. Crown 8vo., pp. 350, cloth, fully illustrated, price 4s.

"The information is presented in the most lucid, graceful, and entertaining manner."—*Economist*.

"Every one who peruses them will be grateful to the author. The history of those creatures whose products become through man's skill so useful to him is given with such charming feeling that the interest of the reader is attracted and enchained, whether he wills or no."—*Era*.

Good Condition.
A Guide to Athletic Training. For Amateurs and Professionals. By C. J. MICHOD, late Secretary to the London Athletic Club. Small 8vo., price 1s.

Dr. Lankester on Food.

A Course of Lectures delivered at the South Kensington Museum. By E. LANKESTER, M.D., F.R.S., F.L.S. New Edition. Price 4s.

"That he has a facility of rendering technical and scientific matters popular this publication abundantly testifies. . . Practical information of this kind cannot but be generally useful, and much of it is contained in these interesting lectures."—*Morning Post.*

"If the mass of the people knew what they eat, what they should eat, and how and by what the human frame is nourished, the sum of human happiness and longevity might be materially increased . . . Full of sound science, curious anecdote, and quaint illustration. Dr. Lankester has a singular power of illustrative keenness, and in the discursive lessons which he delivers on so many subjects there is an overflowing wealth of minute collateral information, which is always brought to the level of the last achievements of science."—*Lancet.*

"Dr. Lankester's style is so facile and attractive that we know of no writer more capable of bringing dry subjects before the public mind in an acceptable form than himself. Many, therefore, who open this volume will be carried away by the pleasure of perusal into a study of useful facts, which they little dreamt of troubling themselves about and would naturally rather shrink from."—*Era.*

In the Plain and on the Mountain.

A Guide for Pedestrians and Mountain Tourists in the Plain and on the Mountain. By CHARLES BONER, author of "Chamois Hunting in Bavaria," "Forest Creatures," &c. With Illustrations of Dress Requisites, &c. Fcap. 8vo., price 1s.

"A little book which compresses into a very small space a great deal of good advice."—*Pall Mall Gazette.*

"We recommend Mr. Boner's book to all travellers, either on mountain or plain."—*Athenæum.*

Mrs. Lankester's Talks about Health.

An explanation of the various process by which life is sustained. Adapted to the understanding of the Young. Small 8vo., price 1s.

LONDON: ROBERT HARDWICKE, 192, PICCADILLY, W.

Royal Humane Society.

INSTITUTED 1774.

To collect and circulate the most approved and effectual methods for Recovering Persons apparently Drowned or Dead, to suggest and provide Suitable Apparatus for, and bestow Rewards on, all who risk their lives in the Preservation or Restoration of Human Life.

SUPPORTED BY VOLUNTARY CONTRIBUTIONS.

Office: 4, Trafalgar Square, Charing Cross.

Patron—THE QUEEN'S MOST EXCELLENT MAJESTY.
Vice-Patron—H.R.H. THE DUKE OF CAMBRIDGE, K.G.
President—HIS GRACE THE DUKE OF ARGYLL, K.T.
Treasurer—T. E. BAKER, Esq.
Secretary—LAMBTON J. H. YOUNG.

Lifeboat Services.

During the Storms of 1863, the Boats of the National Lifeboat Institution saved 417 persons from different wrecks on our coasts. The Institution also expended £13,819. 3s. 2d. in the same period on its Lifeboat Establishments, in addition to granting £1,351. 6s. as rewards for saving 714 shipwrecked persons by its lifeboats and other means.

The Committee of the Institution earnestly APPEAL to the Public for ASSISTANCE to enable them to meet the continued heavy demands on the Institution's 137 Lifeboat Establishments.

Contributions are received by Messrs. Willis & Co., Herries & Co., Coutts & Co., and by all the London and Country Bankers, and by the Secretary, Richard Lewis, Esq., at the Institution, 14, John Street, Adelphi.

www.ingramcontent.com/pod-product-compliance
Lightning Source LLC
Chambersburg PA
CBHW021406230426
43666CB00006B/651